P9-DJL-313

TOP 10

Greatest Lies
About Pregnancy

10. Lamaze Works.

9. Morning Sickness Is Gone by Lunchtime.

8. Good Mothers Love Every Minute of This.

7. You Will Have Your Pre-pregnancy Figure Back in Three Months, Especially If You Nurse.

6. Oil Massages Prevent Stretch Marks.

5. Pregnant Women Have the Most Beautiful Skin and Hair.

4. Exercise During Pregnancy Will Make Your Labor Easier.

3. Pregnancy Brings a Couple Closer Together (Yeah, You and Your Obstetrician!).

2. "From the Back, You Can't Even Tell You're Pregnant!"

1. Pregnancy Only Lasts Nine Months.

The Girlfriends' Guide to Pregnancy

Second Edition

Vicki Iovine

POCKET BOOKS

NEW YORK LONDON TORONTO SYDNEY

The author of this book is not a physician and the ideas, procedures, and suggestions in this book are not intended as a substitute for the medical advice of a trained health professional. All matters regarding your health require medical supervision. Consult your physician before adopting the suggestions in this book, as well as about any condition that may require diagnosis or medical attention. The author and publisher disclaim any liability arising directly or indirectly from the use of the book.

 POCKET BOOKS, a division of Simon & Schuster, Inc.
1230 Avenue of the Americas, New York, NY 10020

Copyright © 1995, 2007 by Vicki Iovine

All rights reserved, including the right to reproduce
this book or portions thereof in any form whatsoever.
For information address Pocket Books, 1230 Avenue
of the Americas, New York, NY 10020

Library of Congress Cataloging-in-Publication Data
Iovine, Vicki.
    The girlfriends' guide to pregnancy / Vicki Iovine.—2nd ed.
      p.   cm.
    Includes index.
    1. Pregnancy.   I. Title.
    RG525.I58 2007
    618.2—dc22   2006051044

ISBN-13: 978-1-4165-2472-4
ISBN-10:   1-4165-2472-X

This Pocket Books trade paperback edition January 2007

10 9 8 7 6 5 4

POCKET and colophon are registered trademarks
of Simon & Schuster, Inc.

Manufactured in the United States of America

Text design by Diane Hobbing of Snap-Haus Graphics

For information regarding special discounts for bulk purchases,
please contact Simon & Schuster Special Sales at 1-800-456-6798
or business@simonandschuster.com

FOR JAMIE, JESSICA, JEREMY, AND JADE

Acknowledgments

1995

Here I am, winner of the life lottery. I have a bunch of kids, a great husband, a new computer (that I sort of know how to use) and *I have written a book,* for heaven's sake! What's left for me now, except perhaps rejoining the other mothers in the car pool? I am grateful to so many people for helping me pull this off. My family, of course, tops any list. My kids will probably talk about this book with their therapists in adulthood, but so far they have been ardent supporters. Not only did they provide me with most of my material, but they cut me some slack to write when they really wanted me at karate practice or the school Christmas pageant. Only a man with my husband Jimmy's confidence and sense of humor could take the beating I occasionally give his gender. Only a man who really had faith in me could believe that I could write a book, raise our kids, and remodel the house with one hand tied behind my back. And only a man who really loved me could never once ask me to cook him dinner during the entire process. I love my family so much that, when I think of them, I can't quite catch my breath.

Before there was the Iovine family, there was the McCarty family, and they are as responsible for this book's happening as anyone. First there is my father, who, in his soul, is really the writer of the family, and my stepmother, Linda, who has been loving me and covering for me since I was twelve. Then there is my mother, who in her soul is really Lucille Ball and who showed me candor and humor in their most uncontrollable forms. And there is my beloved brother, Gregg, who is really my first baby. He always thought his big sister could accomplish anything, and he uncomplainingly allowed me to hone my mothering skills on him. It was he I fed cat food to during *Captain Kangaroo,* and it was he I almost convinced to drink water out of the toilet in my new plastic tea set. It was for him that I beat up a neighborhood kid who teased him for wearing saddle shoes. (See, I told you my mother had a good sense of humor.)

Then there were the people who stood behind me and pushed when my energy or self-confidence failed. They start with my friend of so many years and adventures Bobby Shriver, who has always gotten a kick out of encouraging me to do ridiculous things. He introduced me to Bob Bookman, who was kind enough to laugh at my jokes and help me find the perfect agent. He was assisted in this task by Angela Janklow Harrington, who appropriately got pregnant with her first daughter during this process. Then there is that perfect agent Angela and Bob found for me, Cynthia Cannell, who with her calm and sweet manner (that belied her ability to be a tough advocate if the need arose) actually made me believe I could string more than five words together, and who became a Girlfriend in the process. She also introduced me to the funniest (but not funnier than I) and smartest editor in the world, Dona Chernoff. With that, the Matriarchy was formed. We three mothers were on a rampage, and this book reflects our combined point of view. No day seems complete without a nice long kvetch with each of them on the phone.

I deeply and lovingly thank all my Girlfriends for sharing their stories (and for letting me tell their stories to complete strangers) and for being part of every decision I make every day, from writing this book to cutting my hair to deciding whether it's time for plastic surgery. I cherish our alliance and interdependence. I also love our birthday parties.

I have no false pride that I completed this endeavor alone. It could not have happened without my assistant, Frances Tsow. When she wasn't busy proofreading or numbering the pages of a manuscript that changed several thousand times, she was making sure my kids didn't miss their dentist appointments and organizing their playdates. Best of all, she knew when I needed to take a break (or risk accidentally erasing my manuscript from the computer), when to run out and surprise me with an extralarge iced coffee, or when to just stand back and laugh at the chaos.

I am eternally grateful and endlessly excited, and I look forward to the day when I can walk into a bookstore and see this book (with my name on it, no less) on the shelf.

Acknowledgments
2007

It's been twelve years since the first edition of *The Girlfriends' Guide to Pregnancy* was released. Its success has been nothing short of shocking, but I'm most moved by the personal and sweet connections that the readers and I have developed. When I meet women who have had their babies with this book as their Girlfriend—they oftentimes come up to meet me in a mall, during a book signing or even via my husband's office—they tell me their pregnancy and birth stories. Best of all, they show me pictures of their babies. I can't describe how much I love this and how humble it makes me feel. I love those babies, too.

One of the first people who helped pave the way for this second edition of the book was Tom Freston, former Co-Chairman of Viacom, and a constant friend and mentor to our family. Tom, I will never forget your kindness and I thank you every day when I sit down before a blank computer screen. Next on board with the encouragement to go back to the well, so to speak, and reappraise every word and attitude from a decade of hindsight and experience was Jack Romanos of Simon & Schuster. He was there in 1995 when I had this idea for a little book for pregnant women and, in spite of the impression I had that his interest in personal female stuff was neutral or worse, Jack, you encouraged and supported me in being my outrageous and outraged self. I will always be happy to be "home" at Pocket Books and Simon & Schuster.

Micki Nuding is my new editor at Pocket Books, and it is a match that could come only from the perfect stew of humor, estrogen, shared experience and appreciation for the profound gift we Girlfriends have in each other. Micki, on a personal level, I particularly treasure the freedom you gave me in having my say; in fact, you often encouraged me when I got a little timid.

And winning the No BS Award for Working Writers is my literary agent, Dan Strone, at Trident Media. Dan, you have been so generous in your support and your "Stick to the facts, ma'am" approach that has helped me keep my drama in check. You and Lili have been available to me 24/7, even when I came to you encumbered with some restrictions and old business. Your generosity is much appreciated and your finesse legendary.

I sit in my office in my backyard with my friend and assistant, Jody Leib. Jody has protected me and my time and kept me straight for most of the twelve years since the first edition of this book came out. She is the Queen of the Calendar for our entire family and she keeps my career and family moving forward harmoniously (most of the time). As the old Monty Python skit went, "She's strict, but she's fair." I could never do any of this without you, Jodes. You are a treasured Girlfriend and I love you.

I've dedicated this book to my four kids, who are all teenagers now. That will be my next book, of course. They find me vaguely humiliating most of the time, but they seem proud when yet another one of their teachers is pregnant and in need of *The Girlfriends' Guide*. I think they're most proud of the picture of them as babies on the first inside cover.

My last, and deepest, acknowledgment goes to the Big Daddy, my partner for twenty-five years and, yes, I confess, the catcher of most of my pitched zingers, my true love, Jimmy. Jimmy is the best storyteller in our family, and it's been his keen humor and willingness to give me a character to butt up against that have made my writing career. He may feel at times like Howard Stern's first wife, but he has such an amazing generosity of spirit that he lets me fly. Jimmy, I am the luckiest girl in the world to have met you, and that you trusted me enough to join me in making a family together. You are our family's safe place and I love you dearly. T.N.

Contents

Foreword

Welcome to the Sorority

Pregnant, huh? Well, come on in and sit here beside me, because there is nothing I like more than a woman who is about to have a baby. In fact, just about every mother I know feels the same way. Being pregnant is a time of such anticipation and optimism and dreaming . . . and fear and insecurity and self-doubt (but more about that later). The world loves a pregnant woman, because we all want to protect you and encourage you, and other women who have had babies are ecstatic to have a new member joining our ranks.

In any gathering of women, a camaraderie exists among those who have experienced childbirth. It's like a secret handshake or an ultraviolet mark that only we know, that distinguishes us as veterans of the same war. Complete strangers can bond in ten minutes in a ladies' room sharing the grisly details of their labors. A pregnant woman such as yourself is a probationary member of this sorority. You will be included in all bonding sessions, and you will be embraced and guided by all the other members. And after this forty-week (more or less) probationary period will come the magic time when you will become a charter member, when you have passed the ultimate hazing ritual: DELIVERY.

For the rest of your life you will feel a kinship with the other mothers of the world. You will learn to appreciate each other as only someone who has had a baby can. This sorority of women is full of all sorts of self-congratulation, because only another mother knows what each of us has gone through to qualify for membership. Like veterans of a war, we show our battle scars like medals: cesarean sections, stretch marks, our inability to sneeze without wetting our pants! This is one of the few places where mothers can exhale and stop holding their tummies in. We may weep uncontrollably at kindergarten Christmas pageants, and we may not be able to stay awake past nine o'clock, even on a weekend. But secretly we know, we are earth's real heroes.

I gave birth to four children in six years, two boys and two girls with no twins in the lot, and the lesson I learned (aside from not to trust the rhythm method) is this: 90 percent of the information I needed to get me through these pregnancies came from my Girlfriends who had already had children. Sure, there are a lot of books about pregnancy that you can read. Good student (and terrified person) that I was, I bought them all and read most of them. (By the way, you will probably do the same thing: buy every book on the shelf pertaining to pregnancy and then read the ones that don't confuse, frighten, or depress you, leaving you with this one.) In fact, I now know so much about the technical aspects of this pregnancy business that I am certain that I could deliver *your* baby, even by cesarean section, with nothing but my eyebrow tweezers and newspaper to swaddle the little tyke in, on the floor of a speeding taxi. I know all the exotic terms such as *Braxton Hicks contractions, placenta previa,* and *fundus.*

But the experience of pregnancy is so much more than medical; it is emotional, physical, and social, and I never found a book, in seven years of searching, that addressed those aspects of the experience in the way a good, experienced, and, most important, *candid* Girlfriend could. None of these books ever really seemed to capture the essence of *my* pregnancies. They were too detached, too calm, too neat, too *moderate* for what I was experiencing. To me, pregnancy is an alarming, charming, sloppy, and sentimental affair. Phrases like *momentary discomfort* and *tender to the touch* come nowhere near describing what a procedure like amniocentesis feels like or what newly pregnant breasts feel like. *Sensitive* or *moody* are really lame descriptions of a pregnant woman's emotional life, trust me! When a book told me that I would have a discharge for a few weeks after delivery, I was in no way prepared to be unable to go the four feet from my hospital bed to the bathroom without leaving a grisly trail that looked as if a murder had taken place. No, it was not my beloved doctor or the traditional pregnancy books that prepared me, but rather my Girlfriends. It was my Girlfriends who warned me not to courageously decline my doctor's offer of pain medication after delivery, because after he was home and sleeping in his warm, cushy bed, my epidural would wear off and I would be in my hard, little hospital bed with nothing more than a Tylenol for comfort. It was also my Girlfriends who reassured me that my husband would still make a good father even if he fainted during ultrasounds and refused to cut the umbilical cord. It was my Girlfriends who told me which outfits made my behind look even fatter than it was or if I was acting unbearably Pregzilla. This pregnancy business knocked me broadside at times, and it was usually my Girlfriends who propped me back up.

"But," you are saying to yourself, "I have a wonderful doctor to tell me everything I'll need to know about having a baby." What turnip truck did you just fall off of? Doctors are among my favorite people on earth—in fact, I pray that at least one of my children gets into medical school someday—but I rarely asked my doctor the questions that really mattered to me. Sometimes I was afraid of wasting his time; how could I bother him with endless questions about the earliest point at which I could get an epidural, when there were women in his practice with *real* problems? Sometimes I was afraid to reveal how indelicate and, perhaps, unattractive I often felt I was becoming; for some reason I was completely unconcerned about this man touching my cervix, and yet I withered at the prospect of asking him why I had found a hair growing from my nipple one morning. Often my questions weren't really medical in nature, such as, "Why can't I fit into vintage jeans made for pregnant gals?" and I was paralyzingly afraid of looking as stupid as I felt. After all, having babies is so natural and common that women must be *born* knowing what to do, right? You will be amazed at the things you do not know! If I had called my doctor every time I had a question about pregnancy, he would have been on the phone with me two to three hours a day, and at least half an hour in the middle of the night after I had gotten up to pee for the fifth time.

The Girlfriends' Guide to Pregnancy is the book I'd always hoped to find when I was pregnant. It is the compilation of the experiences, opinions, concerns, complaints, and remedies that my Girlfriends and I had when we were pregnant. If any real medical information is passed along in this book, it is largely accidental, for I leave that domain to the doctors. Desperate as you may be at this point in your life for someone to tell you what to do, I would feel a whole lot better if you would run any of my suggestions by your doctor before adopting them. Think of this book as the jumping-off point for some interesting and informative conversations with your obstetrician. In fact, if there is anything you are too embarrassed to ask him or her, just mark the page in *The Girlfriends' Guide* that discusses it and ask him or her to take a look. You should feel free to disregard or disagree with any part of this book. For example, if you are one of the blessed ones who never experience one single gag of nausea during the nine months of your pregnancy, go ahead and ignore the parts that deal with morning sickness. Just don't talk too much about your good fortune. A safe rule of thumb is: BE CAREFUL NOT TO GET SMUG BECAUSE THE GODS OF PREGNANCY ARE USUALLY FAIR. In other words, if you don't get morning sickness, you will probably be cursed with uncontrollable gas.

We have all heard of women who do pregnancy perfectly. You know the type: a model or actress who is reverently portrayed in women's magazines with bouncing hair and hip outfits with accessories that match. Or *worse,* she is the daughter of your mother's best friend, so you have to hear about and be compared with her every single day. She gains the recommended twenty to twenty-five pounds, her skin stays clear and rosy, she prepares for birth by listening to meditation tapes, she has her own custom seat for her spinning class and cycles up until she is about six centimeters dilated, and she swears she has never felt better in her life. She also has a mate who thinks she is at her most beautiful when swollen with child, who actually *asks questions* at the childbirth preparedness classes, and who, after the baby is born, takes the placenta home and buries it beneath an old oak tree.

This Book Is Not for These Women

It is for the rest of us; those of us who put on twenty pounds between the home pregnancy test and the first doctor's visit. It is for those of us who get our first case of acne since the homecoming dance. It is for those of us who have hemorrhoids so bad that we have considered never eating solid food again, in hopes of avoiding another bowel movement for the rest of our lives. It is for those of us who have considered murdering our partners in their sleep because we thought we heard them say "Moo" when we were getting dressed. It is for those of us who can no longer watch a Pampers commercial without being moved to tears, and who feel it is our responsibility to memorize the faces of children on *America's Most Wanted* so that we can reunite them with their bereft parents.

In other words, this book is for *every* pregnant woman, because I believe that any woman who tells you that her pregnancy is, without exception, the most pleasant and fulfilling time of her life is either lying or has a personality disorder. Besides, I'll bet good money that during their pregnancies, even some of those models and actresses got hemorrhoids.

A Brief History of Girlfriends and Pregnancy

Simply put, having babies is women's work. Until about seventy years ago, men were there for conception and then for the congratulations and the passing out of cigars, but they had precious little to do with what happened in the nine months in between. (Speaking of nine months, let's get one thing straight right now: Pregnancy lasts an average of forty weeks, and by my calculations that equals *ten* months of pregnancy. You may say, "But who's counting?" And I reply vehemently, "*You* will be!" And you will be confused the whole damn time. Are you six months pregnant because you have not seen your period for twenty-four weeks? But that means you have sixteen weeks left. See, there's that ten-month figure again. After you have been without periods for twenty-four weeks, are you "six months pregnant" or "in your seventh month"? God, the whole countdown gave me a headache. All I know for certain is, it didn't go as fast as I hoped it would.)

Anyway, when a woman found out she was pregnant, she naturally turned to the other women of her tribe—her mother, sisters, aunts, and friends—for guidance because, as common as pregnancy is, no first-timer has any idea what the heck is going on when it happens to her. And women who have had children are always more than happy to share their wisdom with the uninitiated.

In those days, doctors were still busying themselves with trying to cure malaria and sewing up farmers who had fallen into their threshing machines, and there was precious little medical business related to pregnancy. The more experienced women of the social group assisted the dumbfounded novice by telling her what to expect, by advising her how to stay as comfortable as possible during the pregnancy and, most important, by reassuring her that her experiences were normal. Since nothing about pregnancy feels in the least bit normal, this was cherished advice. Of course, there was also a lot of passing of what I call "hoodoo wisdom" (you know, those sixth-sense, intuitive, hocus-pocus "truths" that some believe in with all their hearts), such as dangling wedding bands over the pregnant woman's stomach to determine if she was having a boy or a girl, or putting a knife underneath the labor bed to cut the pain—but we have tried to sift through that kind of information in this *Girlfriends' Guide.*

Now doctors usually run the show, except for those fringe people who are willing to face delivery without a neonatal unit next door and a full-time anesthesiologist in residence. Remember all those old Westerns when the poor women died in childbirth? You almost never hear about that happening anymore, thanks to God, clean water, and the American Medical Association. In addition to protecting our babies' lives and our own, doctors monitor our pregnancies and tell us whether there is too much protein in our urine, or if we are at risk for gestational diabetes or some other such tribulation. And let's not forget my personal favorite: Doctors promise to stand between you and calamity during the high drama of labor and delivery.

It is never my intention to undermine the role of doctors in any way, and I would be forever relieved if you would think of this book as a "supplement" of sorts to the serious advice and counsel of your obstetrician. With that burden of guilt and responsibility removed, I would like to say that I believe that women learn some of the most valuable things about pregnancy from other women. Not only were my Girlfriends endlessly giving of their experience and knowledge, but they constantly reassured me that I was normal, and that was surely the greatest gift of all. While every woman believes her pregnancy is unique and special (especially if it is her first), she also yearns to be told that she is no more confused, insecure, or neurotic than the rest of us mothers.

The only problem is that we are a mobile society and we no longer stay within our "tribes." Or as my Girlfriend Kelly's grandmother used to say, "We don't always grow in the garden where we were planted." That means that your mother, aunts, sisters, and experienced Girlfriends may not be around to help you when you get pregnant, because you live in San Diego and they live everywhere from Duluth to Staten Island to St. Petersburg. And, if you are like most women who have not yet had children, you have been spending your time at a job for the years preceding your pregnancy, instead of bonding with the other women in the neighborhood over potluck dinners and butter churning. Millions of us wouldn't know our next-door neighbors if we ran over them in our driveways. So that pretty much leaves you alone with your partner (which is the same as totally alone, in this particular situation) to navigate the choppy waters of pregnancy.

Even if your mother is nearby when you are pregnant, you will soon learn something critically important: EACH GENERATION HAS ITS OWN SET OF PREGNANCY RULES, AND OUR MOTHERS' RULES ARE NOT OURS. For example, our mothers were free to enjoy a cocktail when they felt like it. Nowadays a woman can't go into a restaurant without seeing a warning plaque on the wall connecting fetal alcohol syndrome to a nice cabernet with dinner. Even smoking wasn't the reproductive felony it is now, which was particularly "helpful" because our moms had something nonfattening to put in their mouths to help them avoid gaining more than the fifteen pounds that their doctors prescribed, unlike some of us who reached for jelly beans about once every six minutes.

You will also learn from talking to your mother that the experience of pregnancy, intense as it is while you are going through it, is gradually forgotten almost entirely, as are entire episodes of your babyhood. It sounds absolutely impossible to you now, doesn't it? But you can test it for yourself. Show your mother a baby picture of you and one of your brother or sister, and ask her to tell you who is who. Chances are, she will really have to think about it or use unfair indicators such as the model of the car in the background or the style of her hair. (Make a mental note to yourself now to mark every baby photo that comes into your house as soon as it arrives, because Mommy Alzheimer's is ferocious.)

I occasionally asked my mother things about how it was when she was pregnant with me, and she really only seemed to recall two things: She craved chocolate peanut clusters, and her water broke on the floor of Sears when she was shopping for my layette. Oh, yes, and she told me she sneaked a cigarette in the hospital bathroom to help get her bowels going because she couldn't get discharged until she had had a "movement."

If you mention such concerns as whether to get an amniocentesis or whether you should stop using the microwave to avoid exposing the fetus to some sort of radiation, your mother will look at you as though you are the biggest chump in town, listening to New Age medical mumbo jumbo. She will probably say something like "Honey, you have *got* to relax. When I was pregnant with you, I just went on with my life. You kids *think* too much about everything. Do what you like—the baby will be fine. But for God's sake, you've got to stop eating, because you're beginning to look like the side of a barn."

Needless to say, this is not welcome advice in a generation of women raised to analyze and understand everything from their comfort zones to their G-spots. Add to that the current wave of insanity gripping our nation—the desire to be perfect at everything we do at home and at work—and you can have a substantial group of women in need of some real support. This book is just what the doctor ordered. *The Girlfriends' Guide to Pregnancy* provides the reassurance, advice, and road signs that are invaluable to a pregnant woman.

It will also come in handy for all the fathers-to-be who are convinced that their lovely mates have been taken over by the Body Snatchers. You will learn the fundamental rule of parenthood, which begins with pregnancy: You don't have to be a perfect mother, just good enough. We Girlfriends have absolutely no doubt that you will be more than good enough, and we are here to see to it that you keep your sanity and sense of humor along the way.

TOP 10

Reasons to Suspect You're Pregnant

10. Your Breasts Are Bigger, Puffier, and a Lot More Sensitive.

9. You Need to Urinate Frequently, Especially in the Middle of the night.

8. You're Even More Exhausted Than Usual.

7. Phantom Menstrual Cramps—You Swear Your Period Is About to Start Any Minute.

6. You're Dizzy and Light-Headed and You May Even Faint.

5. nauseous? We're Talking Morning, noon, and night Sickness.

4. The World Begins to Smell Strange and You Think You Could Freelance with Police Dogs to Sniff Out Drugs and Explosives.

3. Feel as If You're Losing Your Mind or Control of Your Emotions? Could Be Pregnancy Insanity.

2. You May Think no Period Is a Telltale Sign, but for You Irregular Gals It's Often not Your First Clue.

1. World-Famous Women's Intuition. Many Girlfriends Swear They Knew They Were Pregnant at the Moment of Conception.

The Girlfriends' Guide to Pregnancy

1

So, What Makes You Think You're Pregnant?

QUITE OFTEN NATURE provides us with physical clues that might make us suspect we are pregnant, even before modern science confirms it. Usually when you find out that you are, indeed, pregnant, you say to yourself with a sudden awakening, "Oh, so *that's* why my . . ." (Fill in the symptom: "boobs hurt"; "bladder fails"; "partner drives me crazy.") Especially in retrospect, you will see that there are usually abundant physical changes to inform you in no uncertain terms that you are pregnant. That is why I am always cynical when I read those stories about unsuspecting women giving birth to babies in airplane bathrooms after nine months of not knowing they were pregnant. Come on now! Most eight-month-old fetuses kick and tumble so fiercely that you can watch your abdomen go from round to nearly square. And what about that inevitable weight gain? Who are these women trying to kid? Either they are trying for the Immaculate Conception excuse or they are just not really paying enough attention to themselves. There are plenty of other changes that, when put together, might lead you to suspect that you are pregnant long before you confirm it with a pregnancy test. What follows is a list of the common early-warning signs.

Breasts

One of the most common changes in the pregnant woman's body is in her breasts. The newly pregnant woman often gets the same puffy breasts that she gets premenstrually, but the consensus among the Girlfriends is that these breasts are a lot more *sensitive*. In fact, taking a shower can be agonizing if you face the stream of water, sleeping on your stomach becomes unbearable, and if your partner should happen to touch your breasts, you will feel completely justified in hitting him with the bedside lamp. Not only are they sensitive and sore, but they are getting bigger and bigger every day. The good news, especially for those of us who have always secretly longed to be big, busty gals, is that they will continue to grow, and they will eventually stop hurting. In a month or so, you and your guy will have a nice new set of playthings.

Peeing

Another symptom that the Girlfriends found in early pregnancy was the need to urinate *a lot*. You may find yourself getting up two or three (or more) times a night to pee, when you used to sleep all night long without even hearing a peep from your bladder. Since fatigue is often another early sign of pregnancy, you will probably learn to loathe all of these interruptions of your precious slumber. Some old folk wisdom says that all this getting up and down all night to pee is nature's way of preparing you for early motherhood, when the up-and-down drill is much the same. I happen to think that this folk wisdom is incorrect, because you will start being able to sleep again later in your pregnancy, and everyone knows a pregnant woman cannot be expected to remember something that she learned six months earlier. Heck, she probably can't remember what happened *yesterday*.

All these nighttime trips can indeed be annoying, but it's usually not as bad as it sounds because almost all of us Girlfriends discovered that we could get out of bed, walk to the bathroom, pee, wipe, walk back to bed, and crawl in, all without opening our eyes one single time. Some of us could even take a drink of water without looking. I, however, was almost always hungry at night, and I frequently ended up in the kitchen after one of my nocturnal pees. If the trip downstairs hadn't awakened me, the refrigerator light was sure to.

Exhaustion

The tiredness of a newly pregnant woman is like a heaviness or being on nighttime cold medication permanently. My Girlfriend Becky, who sells real estate, was so tired that she fell asleep in the car every single time she went to houses of prospective clients. Fortunately for Becky, she had a partner who did most of the driving. The newly pregnant woman may find herself at work unable to think of anything but lying down. My Girl-friend Rosemary used to lock her office door and nap on her sofa for a few minutes every day. Those of us who are fortunate enough to actually take a nap, sleep like the dead, waking up with blanket creases on our faces, red cheeks, and bedhead hair—and usually little more refreshed than we were before. Forget about settling in for a cozy night of watching TiVo'd shows with your honey. You will be snoring before it's time to fast-forward through a commercial. This fatigue can also lead to an inability to stay awake long enough to have sex. Please hand this book to your partner right now.

ATTENTION, PARTNERS OF NEWLY PREGNANT WOMEN:
DO NOT TAKE IT PERSONALLY WHEN YOUR MOMMY-TO-BE WOULD RATHER SLEEP THAN SLEEP WITH YOU! SHE REALLY CAN-NOT HELP IT, AND IT IS ABSOLUTELY NO REFLECTION ON YOUR UNDENIABLE ATTRACTIVENESS OR HOW MUCH SHE LOVES YOU. TRY AGAIN TOMORROW MORNING AFTER SHE HAS HAD SOME REST. (UNLESS, OF COURSE, SHE HAS MORNING SICKNESS, TOO, IN WHICH CASE, TRY THE INTERNET—JUST KIDDING!)

Crampiness

Phantom menstrual cramps can be another sign of pregnancy. Many Girl-friends have never been more certain that their periods were going to start than when they were pregnant. Pregnancy and serious PMS (which is al-ways serious) have several similarities, such as lower-back pressure and that slightly crampy feeling you get right before your period starts. Since I was always paralyzed with the fear that I might miscarry (which, by the way, I never did), I really hated the feeling that my period might start at any minute. I can't count the number of times I felt a little trickle and dropped everything to fly to the bathroom to see if my period had begun.

As you will soon learn, in pregnancy a lot of trickling is going on, as your body goes into overdrive in the vaginal-secretion department.

With all four of my children, I did experience some bleeding early in the pregnancies, and while this is not particularly common, it may happen to you. A general rule of thumb is that if the blood is brownish with no clots and doesn't fill more than one or two sanitary pads, everything is probably all right. If the bleeding is bright red or has clots in it, call your doctor right away. And if there is cramping with the bleeding, call your doctor immediately and ask whether she wants to meet you at her office or the nearest hospital.

Believe me, I know how hysterical you can feel if you are pregnant and you find blood in your underwear, but if it makes you feel any better, all four times my bleeding was bright red (but without cramps), and my doctor just had me rest with my feet up for a couple of days until it went away. My pregnancies were just fine after that. It is perfectly natural to call your doctor for reassurance, but it's not *always* a call for alarm.

Dizziness

Quite a few of my Girlfriends said that they were light-headed early in their pregnancies. Getting out of bed too quickly could give them tunnel vision and make them see stars. Bending over to tie their shoes could result in their having to lie on the floor until the blood returned to their head. A word of caution here: A significant number of women have gotten pregnant after too much to drink, and sometimes pregnancy and a hangover are hard to tell apart. The general rule should be that a hangover that lasts for more than a couple of days could be pregnancy, and it might be a good idea to give up the partying until you know for certain. Even if you aren't pregnant, if you have hangovers that last more than a couple of days, it is probably a good idea for you to give up partying anyway. If you are light-headed, it is usually nothing to worry about, but you could pass out and bonk your head on something, so move slowly and let your blood pressure adjust at its new, slower pace.

Nausea

Nausea is the Waterloo for many newly pregnant women, and it can strike at any point in the pregnancy, usually at the two-month point. They either will find themselves eating everything in sight in a desperate attempt to make the queasiness go away, or they will gag at the mere thought of certain foods. You would think that a nauseous woman is a woman who cannot eat a crumb. Not true. Many of my pregnant Girlfriends experienced starving and vomiting almost simultaneously. Pregnancy can create a gnawing uneasiness in the tummy that is most easily compared to seasickness, and, as with seasickness, food is the only thing that can settle your stomach. The catch is that not *all* food is friendly food. The challenge is in finding just the right foods to soothe the nausea—because you will be amazed at how many of the old favorites, such as cheese, fish, broccoli, or chicken, now make your stomach lurch uncontrollably when you imagine eating them.

Some of my more unfortunate Girlfriends have had such extreme nausea that they would gag right in the middle of a sentence. My poor Girlfriend Maryann was so plagued by morning sickness that she would throw up spontaneously. There would be no warning signs, such as a wave of nausea or a watering of the mouth. One moment she would be chatting normally, and the next minute it was the pea-soup scene from *The Exorcist.* She just sat as quietly as possible with her mouth clenched tightly to try to keep the mess to a minimum. Occasionally, a pregnant woman suffers so much from vomiting, a condition called hyperemesis, that she is hospitalized to keep her hydrated and as comfortable as possible. This unfortunate pregnancy "side effect" isn't usually threatening to the baby, but it can send the mommy right around the bend. As the saying goes, "This, too, shall pass."

Then again, many other Girlfriends have never experienced a gurgle of nausea. This diversity is just another example of how nature gets a kick out of keeping us guessing and never letting us completely relax.

There is really no rhyme or reason in this area of food preferences and sensitivities. You might be like my Girlfriend Sondra, who, when she was pregnant, craved anything spicy. She would start her days with Mexican food drowning in salsa. By lunchtime she was begging her friends to go to sushi bars with her so that she could nibble on the wasabi, even if she couldn't eat the raw fish. (Little microbes might be transmitted from sushi into your intestines, Girlfriends, or your doctor may worry about too much mercury collecting in your body. Just ask your trusted professional for her appraisal of the risk.) Or you might be like my Girlfriend Shannon, who craved "comfort" foods such as mashed potatoes, cereals, and white toast. My Girlfriend Corki got on a fruit kick and lived for straw-berries and nectarines, with a little chocolate thrown in every now and then for variety.

Obviously, the goal is to eat some foods from the five major food groups, if not at every meal, then at least once a day. DO NOT PANIC, HOWEVER, IF YOU FAIL TO EAT TEXTBOOK BALANCED MEALS EVERY DAY DURING YOUR FIRST COUPLE OF MONTHS OF PREGNANCY. At least one recent study indicated that food aversions are actually nature's way of protecting you from certain risky foods. So, if you would rather lick dirt than eat broccoli, maybe your body just isn't ready to process that particularly aggressive food. No matter how vehement those other pregnancy books are about your needing eight ounces of protein, four glasses of milk, and a bushel of green, leafy vegeta-bles every day, just do the best you can and KEEP TALKING TO YOUR DOCTOR. He or she may prescribe vitamin supplements to help carry you through the nauseous period and into the second trimester, when you will be thrilled to eat nearly anything that is placed before you. You may find that a calcium pill is as effective as the glass of milk that makes your eyes water and your throat close down. The bottom line this early in your suspected pregnancy is this: If you feel "green" and you haven't got a tem-perature, it's time for a pregnancy test.

Note: If you crave nonfood items, such as the above-mentioned dirt or paint chips (and some pregnant women do), avoid the urge and call your doctor TODAY.

Sensitivity to Odors

For a lot of women, including myself, the first sign that they are pregnant is that the world begins to smell strange. Common aromas seem to get more powerful or cloying. My Girlfriend Mindy developed such an aver-sion to the smell of dairy products when she was pregnant that she couldn't walk into a grocery store or a delicatessen for fear of smelling the cheese and throwing up in the aisle. One morning she saw me pouring cream into my coffee and started making noises like a cat trying to get up a hair ball. Continuing with this cat theme, my Girlfriend Lynn had to beg her husband to take over the feeding of their cat because the first whiff of the Seafood Surprise when the can was opened sent her streaking for the sink.

By the way, if you do have a cat, and you are indeed pregnant, it is time to give another member of the household the job of changing the cat litter. Ask your doctor for details, but cat poopoo can give some virus to pregnant women, so steer clear of it (as if I have to twist your arm, right?).

During my first pregnancy, I was so certain that my bed pillows and comforter were mildewed that I wrapped them in plastic garbage bags and disposed of them. I immediately (and irrationally, according to my husband) replaced the pillows and comforter with brand-new ones, only to discover when I crawled into bed that night that they smelled exactly the same!

Insanity

Another indication that you might be pregnant can be the feeling that you are losing your mind, or at least some vague control of your emotions. You may feel as though you have a monster case of PMS. This is not something I am proud to share with you, but as your Girlfriend, I will: Two different times, the first doctors to suggest to me that I might be pregnant were not gynecologists, but psychiatrists. One time, my husband calmly put me in the car and drove me to his therapist right after I tried to knock his head off by throwing a book across the room. (Believe me when I say this behavior was not only uncharacteristic of me, it was absolutely unacceptable to him.) Another time, after I tried to steer the car *while my husband was driving* (because he wasn't taking the route I had so generously suggested), I ended up on a therapist's couch sobbing that I feared I was going through early menopause because I just didn't feel like myself and my periods had stopped. That menopause turned out to be my baby Jessica, a possibility that I had not even considered.

Even if you are not prone to violent outbursts, you may experience the hormonal irrationality of pregnancy in the form of weepiness or utter lack of humor. My Girlfriend Amy, who is normally the sweetest of Southern belles, was so cranky when she was pregnant that she actually became funny. The contrast between her usual tiny-blond demeanor and her general pissed-off state during pregnancy was so dramatic that it was comical, not unlike a toddler swearing.

One of the most important things to consider during this time of emotional whiplash (aside from putting off the cleaning of any handguns) is the probability that *you* will be completely unaware of your strange behavior. If your partner or friends dare to suggest to you that maybe you aren't yourself these days, you will certainly feel attacked and unfairly judged (and you will begin formulating plans to have them poisoned). As convinced as you may be of your rationality and of everyone else's irrationality, you really are not normal, and you should just accept it and allow for it. In other words, this is not the time to file for divorce, change your job, buy a house, or, most important, cut your hair.

No Period

You might think that not getting your period is a pretty reliable indication that a bun is in your oven, but that was never my first clue. Sure, millions of women have regular twenty-eight-day cycles and know exactly when to expect their period, right down to whether it will be before breakfast or after dinner. I, however, am all over the place. Not only am I irregular, I am usually too distracted by the business of living to have even a vague notion of when my "friend" (don't you just hate that term?) is coming. I have a hard enough time remembering to fill my car with gas, and it comes equipped with a gauge.

The fun part about this absentmindedness is that it can keep your life full of surprises; one day you wake up expecting the same old routine, and instead you discover you are going to have a baby! The troublesome part of this absentmindedness is that when you do confirm that you are pregnant, your doctor will invariably ask you for the date of your last period, and you will have to either lie (as I have always done) or give some lame answer like "It was the day after they announced the winner on *American Idol.*"

My Girlfriend Mindy had missed two periods before she began to suspect that she might be pregnant. I think that she, like a lot of us, was not particularly upset about missing two weeks of tampons and cramps, so she accepted her lack of periods at face value: *A gift from God.* One thing, though, that I have learned from experience is that it is helpful to have a vague familiarity with your cycle, because the new home-pregnancy tests are so sensitive that you can often know if you are pregnant as early as nine or ten days after *the deed.* And since it only makes sense that you would want to protect your pregnancy from the earliest possible moment, a positive test result could inspire you to stop smoking or drinking or taking Prozac (with medical supervision, of course) immediately.

Intuition

We women are supposedly famous for it, and while it has never happened to me, I have a number of reliable Girlfriends who have never previously claimed to have supernatural powers but who swear they knew they were pregnant the instant it happened. They felt something come over them, like a shudder or an instant awareness that this particular roll in the hay wasn't like all the rest; something momentous had occurred. Scientist (or cynic) that I am, I have asked these women if they have ever felt that mystical sensation and *not* been pregnant and just never mentioned it to anyone. Or if perhaps the event wasn't heightened by their knowing that they were having sex on day fourteen of their twenty-eight-day cycle and they weren't using birth control. (You don't have to be a member of the Psychic Network to know that one out of the five times that you get a sperm to an egg, you make a baby.) But, no, these Girlfriends insist that they felt different physically and psychically from that climax onward. And you know what? I believe them, even if I don't understand or relate to any of it.

If you are feeling any of these symptoms, alone or in groups, and if you don't yet know for certain whether you are pregnant, then what in the world are you reading this book for? No, I'm just kidding. You must have a pretty good hunch that a baby is in your future, so you'd best get in touch with a good obstetrician and start taking special care of your baby and yourself right now.

2

Sharing the Wonderful News

SINCE THE BEGINNING of time, any woman who has gotten pregnant by a man who has a job and is not married to someone else has been congratulated and showered with best wishes. (One would hope that she gets showered with more than just wishes, and I will address a good partner's and a best friend's responsibilities in this area later.) The news that you are pregnant is BIG, each and every time it happens. You know this already by the way you feel when your doctor, nurse practitioner, or any stranger in a white coat comes out of the little lab room with a big smile on his or her face.

The general rule is, if this is your first pregnancy, you will tell your baby daddy the glorious news before you tell anyone else (unless you live in Pine Valley and you are awaiting the DNA reports determining paternity). If this is your second or third baby, however, you will inform everyone on your email list by PDA and text-message the rest. And if this is your fourth or subsequent pregnancy, well, judging by my own experience, it doesn't even pay to mention it until someone asks.

If women and men were really emotional equals, then all prospective fathers would be with the potential mothers, waiting anxiously in the doctor's office for this momentous news. There they would sit with you, flipping through old copies of *Fit Pregnancy* or studying the manuals on the human papilloma virus. If this is your first pregnancy, there is a chance that your partner will indeed be there with you to see the nurse and her smile. But if he's not, remember, perfectly good partners, including my own, are not always with their beloveds when they learn they are pregnant. They can still grow up to be wonderful and attentive fathers. Keep this bit of advice in mind: One good kind of daddy is a daddy with a job, and a daddy-to-be with a job might not be able to get away for an afternoon of sitting in the gynecologist's office. Be pragmatic; a busy man does not automatically equal a bad father. Besides, three home pregnancy tests that came up undeniably positive may be as much excitement as he can take in a week.

Your Obstetrician

At the risk of repeating myself, let me assure you that home pregnancy tests—yes, the standard sticks you pee on and wait for a sign in the little window, or a colored tip to appear, or a stork to fly in your chimney—are virtually always correct if the result is positive. In spite of this, most first-timers do not consider themselves officially pregnant until their doctor tells them so. This is why we call to make an appointment for an office test ASAP! Even if you strongly suspect that you are indeed pregnant, the shock of hearing this news from a medical professional can be so stunning that even the most capable and stouthearted of us become weak and quite grateful that someone familiar with CPR is in the room with us.

Your first response will be the slightly inane question "Are you SURE?" And without a doubt, your next question will be "When is it due?" Few things are more exciting than watching your doctor or practitioner pull out one of those little cardboard wheels with the numbers to compute your baby's expected arrival. No matter how often your Girlfriends advise you not to rely on it too much, you will embrace that date firmly and plan your entire life around it. And when that due date comes and goes with no baby in sight, as it frequently does with women expecting their first babies, you will become a directionless person without the slightest clue how to pass the time until you feel your first labor pain.

By the time I was pregnant with my third and fourth babies, I had boxes of those home pregnancy tests in my medicine cabinet. I routinely took them whenever I was overtired, bloated, burpy, or just bored. What the heck; I'd already spent the money, just in case, and they were a cinch to use as long as I was careful not to pee on my hand. When I finally got a positive result, I was repeatedly so stunned that I immediately reached for another kit to confirm. Here was one of the few times that a pregnant woman's constant need to urinate came in handy. If the results were unanimous, I'd make a note to call my doctor to let him know that I was pregnant *again* and arrange to drop by for a visit in a week or two for some information, such as whether there was a heartbeat (they can often see a little flashing beat as early as six weeks with ultrasound) and whether it was time to start applying to preschools, *again.*

If your mate *is* in the doctor's office with you when you are given the glorious news, the two of you can rejoice together and cry and bury your heads in each other's shoulder, just as those couples do on the TV commercials for home pregnancy tests or fertility clinics. If your partner can't be there with you, you can spend the next couple of minutes being patted and congratulated by the doctor's staff and figuring out the best way to tell your guy that he is going to be a daddy.

Telling "Daddy"

Some of my Girlfriends are quite sentimental about how they share this delicious information. Candlelit meals with romantic music in the background are popular in my crowd, as are clever emails, teddy bears waiting at the front door, or going for a walk together as soon as you both get home. But if my husband were to come home to a setup like that, he would think I had joined a cult and given all our money to the swami. He would be so relieved to hear I was *only* having a baby that my announcement would be anticlimactic.

Having watched far more TV than was good for me, I always imagined telling my husband as we walked hand in hand along the beach at sunset. I would turn to him and he would embrace me and we would look out to sea as we dreamed of our child's future. Perhaps he would even sing "Soliloquy" from *Carousel,* I don't know. Anyway, it never happened. What did happen was usually something like this: I would call him from the doctor's office and hysterically scream at his assistant, "What do you mean, can you take a message? You just tell him to get out of that damn meeting and talk to me right now, because I'm PREGNANT!" Progesterone and I don't get along very well.

I did try the romantic-dinner approach when I learned I was pregnant for the fourth time in six years, and he'd never expressed a desire to have another child after our *first* was born, and I was desperate, and this is what I learned: When you are telling your partner that he is going to be a father and you are looking directly into his eyes, it is almost impossible not to start crying before you even get the first word out. No matter how many times it has happened to you or how comfortable you may be about your new condition, the first couple of times that you say the words "I am going to have a baby," you can hardly form the words because of how much your chin quivers. Maybe it was my terror that he'd pack up and leave me alone with three babies and another on the way, and two dogs and a pregnant feral cat hiding behind the water heater in the garage that viciously scratched any toddler or gardener or mommy who tried to pull her out. Or maybe it was my mushiness over all things having to do with romance and babies (it was years later that I learned those two things are mutually exclusive, at least for about five years, but I'm digressing here). But I nearly choked to death before I could get beyond "Honey, guess what?" My poor husband imagined all sorts of disasters, such as the dog died or I lost his baseball jacket, before I finally spit out the words "We're gonna have another baby." And when I finally did, his expression seemed to say, "You're not going to play the baby card again, are you?"

As a matter of fact, this last time I distinctly remember him going on to say, "How could you do this to me?" I mumbled something to the effect that my elementary understanding of biology indicated that this was something *he* had done to *me,* but this really wasn't the time to quibble. In fact, now that I think about it, it might have been the time to take all the sharp flatware and heavy glasses off the table between us. Before I dissolved into a puddle of hurt feelings, I recalled that my Girlfriend Mindy's husband had said something equally enthusiastic to her when she had gotten pregnant six years before. I believe his exact response was "I'm sorry, but I'm just not ready." As a matter of fact, he wasn't certain if he was ready for most of her pregnancy and was reading old issues of *Road & Track* while she was in labor for forty hours. But the minute their baby girl took her first breath, he became her devoted slave. A father couldn't love his baby more.

Keep daddies like these in mind, because they both started out slowly and then became candidates for Father of the Decade. It isn't necessarily wise to take a mate's first response much to heart. Sure, these days, guys are theoretically more evolved and more in touch with their nurturing side, but even the guys who claim to feel *their* biological clocks ticking louder than yours, or who mention in a moment of intimacy that they wish *they* could nurse a child, too, can turn into thick foreheads when told they have to parent something. In my case, when my loving husband

Telling Girlfriends

After about the age of twenty-one, any woman's announcement that she is pregnant with the child of any man outside of prison or in rehab is met with great glee. We women don't usually respond by worrying if you two can afford it or if it is too early in your relationship, at least not for long. We just like pregnancy, and rarely do we care about the practical aspects. Those are *your* fish to fry. Your friends who have never had children will welcome it as an enjoyable diversion: spending the next nine months watching you get huge. Your friends with kids will be deeply grateful for the opportunity to share with you every detail of their own pregnancies, especially their deliveries. In fact, one feature of *The Girlfriends' Guide* that you will come to love is your freedom to shut it when you feel that you've had it up to here with pregnancy.

After your Girlfriends know that you are pregnant, you will never again have a conversation with them that doesn't include questions about the baby. Some pregnant Girlfriends start to feel like a vessel rather than a person because their whole identities seem wrapped up in gestating. Other Girlfriends can recount every detail about *their* pregnancies until the listener wants to shoot herself for asking in the first place. Your empathetic Girlfriends will tell you how great you look and how you're hardly putting on any weight. Decide for yourself if you want to believe them. I never did.

Telling Mothers

Telling your mother that you are pregnant can be much more fun than you might initially imagine. This is especially true if your mother can say your partner's name without spitting on the ground or seeking a restraining order. Astonishingly, the further you proceed in your pregnancy, the more pleasant and reassuring it is to be around the very same person who, just months before, inspired you to get caller ID so that you could screen your calls.

This could be the beginning of a beautiful relationship because it is the official transformation from being Mommy's little girl into being another woman, *almost* equal in stature. You, too, are going to be somebody's mother. You might find yourself thinking about the mother you remember from when you were really small, the way she took care of you and the things she said to you. You are already inclined to be sentimental in your hormone-jostled state, and you may suddenly remember things like the way she used to make a trail of jelly beans from your bedroom door to where your Easter basket was hidden so that you really believed the Easter bunny had been there, or the way she always bought you an ice cream cone after a dentist's visit, and you will sob (a response you will find occurring with much more frequency as the pregnancy progresses).

Or something quite the opposite might happen. You might have total recall of every unenlightened move you think your mother ever made raising you, and you could spend your entire pregnancy strategizing how to be as *unlike* her as possible. Several of my Girlfriends got quite panicky at the thought that they were doomed to become their own mother. First of all, remember that there is an element of choice here; you are free to adopt or reject all sorts of models of behavior, including your mother's. Second, and much more valuable, is this advice: Take this time to get to know your mother better, because you will come away with a much more empathetic perception of her. For once in your life, you may understand why she publicly embarrassed you in high school because she caught you riding on the back of a motorcycle. All you have to do is picture your own baby strapped to the back of a Harley with a seventeen-year-old at the wheel to understand her hysteria.

Unless your mother is Joan Crawford, she will always be interested in your condition and deeply concerned for your well-being (even if most of her actual advice will sound inapplicable to birthing in the twenty-first century). If you think that this is kind of nice, just wait until the baby is born. If you are one of the many lucky ones, you will notice that your mother seems to love your baby as much as you do, and that is the beginning of the biggest bond in the world.

Remember, baby daddies have been known to come and go in our society, but once your mother has that lovelock on your kid, she can be a great constant in your child's life. And you will begin to realize that maybe she didn't do as bad a job raising you as you'd thought. Not as good as the job you're going to do, of course, but not bad.

I spend this time talking about mothers for two reasons: First, I want to encourage Girlfriends who still have a mother around to take the necessary steps to allow her to share in this pregnancy. Second, for those of you who have lost your mother, or who have a relationship far too dysfunctional to repair in nine months, I want to speak out in honor of the mother-in-law. Remember, it is *her* baby's baby, too, and she might be just the person for you to bond with. Ignore her meddling in what you eat and whether you should be reaching for anything over your head. (There was an old wives' tale that when you reach over your head, you wrap the umbilical cord around the baby's neck. Forget about it.) Remember, this is a woman who would bite her own arm off to make your little baby more comfortable, OR EVEN BABYSIT IF BEGGED. Even if she doesn't seem all that crazy about you, she will love her son's baby. And if you are a loving mother to her grandchild, she will probably learn to love you, too. Put it this way: If it's ever going to happen, now is the time.

The most reassuring feeling for a mother is to know that she can let her guard down for a few hours, knowing that someone else is looking after her child with the same eagle eye and fierce protectiveness that she would. Babysitters are great, but you can never be sure whether in an earthquake they would remember to pick up your precious baby before sprinting out of the house to save their own life. A grandma would not only pick up the baby, she would make sure to grab the baby book and the antique christening dress (even if she had to trample you to do so). I know for certain that if my mother-in-law witnessed any sort of unkindness to my child on the preschool playground, she would either hit the inattentive teacher or burn the whole school down (but, of course, she's Sicilian).

The Girlfriends' advice pertaining to mothers is simple: LET THEM INTO THIS PREGNANCY. Contrary to all indications, they are not there to judge you or tell you what you are doing wrong in your pregnancy. And if they are, try to overlook it, because that kind of concern and commitment are impossible to find anywhere else.

Telling Your Daddy

Sharing the news with your father can be fun, but it is different from telling your mother. If you and your mate are together when you tell your father, you might feel Daddy's eyes come to rest on him, as if to say, "OK. You got her into this fix, and you better take care of her or I will have to kill you."

Most of my Girlfriends agree that your dad is happy if you are happy, but that, like most men, he doesn't immediately fall into baby rapture;

that happens when the baby actually arrives. Think of it this way: Some people can look at an outfit on a hanger and know just what it will look like on. Other people need to wear the thing for a while before they understand the fit. Same thing with babies: Most men can't imagine fatherhood or grandfatherhood until they are holding the little darlings. You may notice that your father gets nervous if he hears you and your mother talking too much and too graphically about your pregnancy. It is important to remember that it is his job to be suspicious of anything that might hurt you. Remember, this is the guy who wanted to hit a doctor for making you cry when you got stitches, so this alien baby who might be making you vomit uncontrollably or who might take fourteen hours to get out of your body isn't sending your father into a tizzy of planning and daydreaming, as it is you and your mother.

One other little thing about telling your father that you are pregnant: This may be the first time in your entire life that you have boldly declared to him that you are no longer a virgin. I don't know about you, but I managed to live for over thirty years without any overt reference to my sex life in front of my father. Sure, he probably had his suspicions, especially after I started living with my boyfriend in college, but we could still pretend. There is no skirting the sex issue once you announce that you are going to have a baby. Dad's bound to know how that happened, which may be another reason his gaze shifts so quickly to your partner upon hearing the news.

When Should You Tell?

Quite a number of people believe that a newly pregnant woman should not announce her condition until most of the danger of miscarriage has passed, usually at about three months. In fact, if you are Jewish, there are "rules" about not bringing any baby clothes or furniture into the house before the baby is born safe and sound, for fear of jinxing it in some way. Being neither Jewish nor particularly reserved in nature, I have consistently told people I was pregnant from the moment I knew. (But I must admit I felt strange about buying baby clothes or toys before the baby was born, as opposed to furniture and supplies, because they seemed so personal.) It's simply that I cannot keep a secret of that magnitude. I remember sitting at dinner one night with my Girlfriend Patti and a number of other people, blabbing about my new pregnancy with all the self-importance of a woman who had just invented the condition. I so enjoyed being the object of everyone's attention, surrounded by so much concern about whether I was eating enough, and if my chair was comfortable enough. Two months later, Patti told me that she had known that night that she was pregnant, too, but didn't want to tell anyone at the dinner until she was sure the pregnancy was "a keeper." I guess I did feel a little sheepish about glomming all the attention when she was as deserving as I was of tender care and special congratulations. But as my mother says, "It pays to advertise."

If you don't tell your closest friends that you are pregnant, how else do you explain why you no longer have the energy to lift your gym bag, let alone take a ninety-minute pole-dancing class? How else do you explain to your gracious hostess that those capers she so imaginatively tossed into your salad are making your eyes water and your throat spasm? And how else do you excuse yourself to a colleague who has walked into your office and found you asleep with your head on your keyboard? I suppose you could give chronic fatigue syndrome a try, but then how do you explain the newly upholstered look your body is taking on?

People give pregnant women wide berth (literally and figuratively), and it is a universally accepted excuse for all kinds of unforgivable behavior, so I would advise invoking it whenever possible. A word of warning, however: THIS EXCUSE LOSES ITS MAGICAL EFFECT ON YOUR PARTNER WITHIN A COUPLE OF MONTHS, AND IT HAS ABSOLUTELY NO POWER OVER HIM BY THE SECOND PREGNANCY. Your partner will look up from his football game to notice you moving the sofa across the room by yourself and do nothing, while a stranger who sees that you are pregnant won't let you lift your own grocery bags.

Of course, there is a good reason why many women keep their early pregnancy a secret: About 10 percent of all pregnancies end in miscarriage within the first twelve weeks. If such a disaster happens to you, it will undoubtedly add to your grief to have to recount repeatedly your tragedy. I have seen a few of my most cherished Girlfriends beginning to heal from the physical and emotional toll of miscarriage, then having to endure an uninformed person's coming up to them and asking how the baby is doing. It was deeply painful for all concerned. I suppose the solution is to tell only those people who would be puzzled by your bizarre behavior (or anyone who has the gall to suggest that you should consider dieting), and to save the megaphones and skywriters for later in your pregnancy.

Total Strangers

You will be amazed at how easy it is to drop your pregnancy into absolutely any conversation or circumstance. If you are circumspect and have kept mum through the entire first trimester, you will nearly explode with the news right at the three-month mark. That kind of a secret is like rice in a pressure cooker: When it bursts, it flies everywhere. Telling people you are pregnant works like a charm when you want some special treatment, such as permission to move to the front of the line in the ladies' room at the movies, which is very useful if you drink large sodas with your popcorn.

In the beginning, you will have to declare your condition because most people either are not too observant or are deathly afraid of congratulating you on your pregnancy only to learn that you aren't pregnant and have simply been eating your way through the universe. (In fact, you are generally well-advised *never* to congratulate a woman on her apparent pregnancy until she shows you her positive pregnancy test, because if she is not pregnant, you automatically become the bonehead of the universe.) It couldn't hurt to tell everyone from the checkout clerk to the policeman who stops you for speeding that you are in that exceptional state called pregnancy. Who knows—they might offer to bag your groceries or give you a police escort to the nearest clean public restroom. At the least, they will give you a nice smile and a few kind words, which is more than most people give you these days. But be prepared—if the person you are telling has borne a child of her own, you may be in for a never-ending monologue about her labor and delivery. It's sad, but we really can't help ourselves.

The Girlfriends are unanimous in this warning regarding strangers: THEY WILL INSIST ON RUBBING YOUR STOMACH AND THEY WILL NEVER ASK FOR YOUR PERMISSION TO DO SO. If you think that this is going to bother you, you might consider keeping your arms folded protectively in front of you. Don't forget, you are completely entitled to take a step back and announce the No Touching

Rule. It's just that people feel you're not a good sport if you don't allow them to manhandle you. I didn't mind it too much when I was cutely pregnant in the second trimester, but by the end, when I was so pregnant I had corners and my belly button popped completely out like on a Butterball turkey, I really hated people touching me, especially if I didn't even know them.

3

Pregnancy Is a Total Body Experience

BEFORE I BECAME pregnant for the first time, I naively believed that the only part of my body that would be affected would be my tummy. I took great satisfaction that I had always been slim and active, and I knew that I would sail through pregnancy with just an adorable bump of a tummy atop my lean, athletic legs. Yeah, right. When I was pregnant, I was pregnant from my chipmunk cheeks to my water-retaining ankles. The legs I was shaving in the shower looked and felt like those of a stranger, so round and dimply were my knees. If I allowed my arms to lie flat against my sides, they looked as wide as my thighs. (Keep this in mind: Sleeveless and pregnant don't always mix.) My wedding ring didn't spin on my ring finger anymore. And, worst of all, I had cellulite so bad, it looked as if I had been pelted with cottage cheese. It wasn't just me, I swear! I have a Girlfriend who is a professional model (she threatened to tell one of my secrets if I told you her name) who gained so much weight in her face that I didn't recognize her in the restaurant where we were meeting for dinner and I walked right past her. If you are like me, you have loving friends who will reassure you that your face hasn't changed at all, and that from the back you don't even look pregnant. They will say that you look healthier and more beautiful than ever. THEY ARE LYING! Sure, pregnancy is adorable, but if you think it's your best look, just wait until you get your old look back and the compliments start flowing—few people will come up to you and say, "I really miss your bump and big booty."

Let's talk about the concept of gaining weight—how much is too much and how much is too little, and what repercussions it will have on your body for the rest of your young life. I will begin by saying that if you are obese or anorexic, your weight is your own private issue, one for you and your doctor to deal with. I will also say that it should be understood that the baby's health is more important than any other consideration, and that any woman who starves herself or eats only trash foods should permanently be ostracized from the community of Girlfriends, if not from the universe.

That aside, let's talk about the rest of us, those who read in some scolding and terrifying pregnancy book whose name must not be mentioned (like Voldemort's) that the weight gain is supposed to progress something like this: zero to three pounds in the first trimester, ten to twelve pounds during the second trimester, and eight to ten pounds during the third trimester. If we don't match up, we live in dread of the weighing days at the doctor's office. A number of us Girlfriends passed that suggested twenty-five-pound weight gain mark at about the seventh month, just when we are really getting good and hungry. In fact, I have been known to put on so much weight in the first trimester that when the nurse asks me on my first visit what my pre-pregnancy weight was, I lie and add five or ten pounds so that she won't know I have already gained *another* ten pounds.

Pathetically, most women learn to gauge their pregnancy based on what their weight gain was for a particular doctor's appointment. If I had a visit where there was no weight increase since the last visit three weeks ago, I would beam with pride, relief, and self-satisfaction for days. I would call my friends to tell them how the baby was doing, then *casually* mention that I hadn't gained any weight. Then on those visits that I was told I had gained seven pounds in less than a month, I would be so embarrassed and humiliated that I would cry, and I *never* told anyone that I had even seen the doctor, let alone been weighed. After four children I have finally learned two lessons, one vitally important and one just useful. The important lesson is: OUR SELF-ESTEEM ISSUES THAT ARE TIED TO WEIGHT, AND HAVE BEEN SINCE PUBERTY, ARE NEVER MORE INAPPROPRIATE THAN WHEN WE ARE PREGNANT.

Pregnancy is a great time to learn the life lesson of surrender. This body is not for your personal enjoyment at the moment. It is a cozy home in which a child is growing, and you can choose to fight it or to relax and enjoy the ride. *The Girlfriends' Guide* knows how hard it can be for a generation of skinny-worshippers to watch themselves transform in this alarming way, because we all felt that way (except my Girlfriend Sondra, but she never got cellulite, so she shouldn't count). That is why I tell you the straight information and then sit back and laugh with you about it, because your sense of humor may be the only thing to get you through these trying times. My Girlfriend Jill just delivered her first baby a couple of weeks ago, and when I visited her in the hospital, she shared a great insight: No one, except her, ever even thought about her weight gain. They thought she looked lovely and never seemed to analyze the circumference of her knees or upper arms. She was not fat or thin; she was just PREGNANT. And anybody with a heart loves two things: weddings and pregnant women.

The other lesson I learned, the simply useful one, is this: STAND BACKWARD ON THE SCALE WHEN YOU ARE BEING WEIGHED AT THE DOCTOR'S OFFICE AND ASK THEM NOT TO TELL YOU HOW MUCH YOU'VE GAINED OR LOST. Some may cluck and look as if they're about to lecture you on body-image issues, but just cut them off by saying, "There's a betting pool in my family about my total gain, and even I can't know till delivery or my husband will be disqualified." No law says you need to have that information every visit. Trust me: If the doctor looks at your chart and notices a problem, he or she will tell you soon enough. Otherwise, what difference does it really make to you? You are getting heavier—so what? Get over it.

By the way, you might be as secretly gratified as I was to notice that women who are what I call "professionally thin"—meaning that because they are actresses, models, or performers, they *have* to be skinny—often really pack on the pounds during pregnancy. I'm talking sixty to seventy pounds for some of the most svelte women you have ever seen on television or in magazines. It must be the relief of not having to live on rice cakes and cigarettes for nine months. My girlfriend Shannon, who is a gorgeous actress, started each pregnant day with eggs, bacon, and so much white toast that she would go through a loaf every other day. She just had a fabulous time, and after the baby was born, she dieted and worked out until she was thin and fit and even more beautiful than she had been before. That is precisely what the other beauties have done, and you can, too—so go ahead and EAT. Heck, you might as well; you can't get drunk, you can't slink around in a sexy black minidress, you can't even take medicine when you are suffering from a cold. What other joys are there for pregnant women? Besides, society is suspicious of skinny pregnant women because we worry that the baby isn't being properly nourished. Just look at Angelina Jolie's first pregnancy and the uproar the tabloids created with her twiggy arms and legs, and that was *before* she moved to Namibia.

The Upholstered Body

As any good subscriber to PMS already knows, the female body is capable of retaining up to five pounds of completely unnecessary (in my estimation) body fluids. The only relief is the arrival of your period. Unfortunately, when you become pregnant, that period is postponed by about forty weeks. So even before you begin putting on actual "baby weight," you might begin to grow, and you may continue to retain water until you find that your rings are too tight and you have "cankles" (when your calves and ankles have no line of demarcation) by the end of a long day on your feet. Your eyes may look a bit puffy, too. You would think that with all the peeing you are doing, there wouldn't be enough water in your body to make spit, but nature makes sure that no one is going to threaten your precious placental fluid and future milk factory. One Girlfriend used to eat only watermelon for the entire day before her monthly visit to her obstetrician because watermelon is a natural diuretic, and she kept her water weight as low as possible for the loathsome chore of being weighed at each visit. *I am not recommending this to you,* but, hey, a little watermelon every once in a while might help keep the puffiness manageable. My Girlfriend Charlotte offers this tip for keeping some facial swelling down: Put a small block of wood, about an inch thick, under the legs at the head of the bed so that you're sleeping on a slight incline. I ran this by a doctor and he endorsed it, adding that it can also help with the gastric reflux (heartburn) that bedevils many mommies-to-be.

The waistline is the second (after the bustline) biggest noticeable change in early pregnancy. Especially if this is your first pregnancy and your stomach muscles have never been traumatized before, your waistline will *widen* quite a few weeks before your belly starts to look rounded. (If this is your second or a subsequent pregnancy, your belly will pooch out about five minutes after you learn you are pregnant, and in ten minutes you will look five months pregnant.) Imagine a straight line from your armpit to your hips, and you will get the basic idea of what this waist-widening looks like. You won't look fat or pregnant at this stage, but you probably won't be able to button your jeans all the way to the top unless they are very low rise. Skirts and fitted dresses may start to strain, too, so rather than look like a "before" Trim-Fast model, move into bigger sizes or looser styles as soon as you and your zipper begin to wrestle.

The Breasts

Your breasts will also start to change almost immediately. They get bigger, much bigger, and heavier. Those of us who were never particularly buxom look at our newly pregnant breasts wondering if these beauties will stay this big forever, and we silently pray to God that they will. Echoing our prayers are our husbands, who now think that maybe this pregnancy business isn't so bad after all. Sondra's husband, Ray, looks forward to the arrival of what he calls the Titty Fairy with the same enthusiasm most six-year-olds have for the Tooth Fairy.

The good news about the breasts is that they will continue to grow throughout your pregnancy. That aching soreness I talked about in chapter 1 will disappear by the end of the first couple of months. You will really have yourself a nice set of knockers for a while—usually until your stomach gets so big that it dwarfs even your mammoth breasts. The most important bit of Girlfriends' advice regarding pregnant breasts is WEAR A BRA. Don't allow your ripe melons to strain their ligaments at a time like this. Pregnancy and childbirth are hard on breasts, what with all the stretching and swelling and sucking that goes on, and you should coddle them as much as possible.

The bad news is that once you have finished gestating and nursing, you will be left with breasts that look like water balloons that have sprung a small leak. Not only do they not retain their pregnancy lusciousness, they are actually smaller and/or saggier than they were before you got pregnant. I know this is terrible news to give you, and you may want to insist that I don't know what I am talking about and throw this book to the floor. But I have made it my business at every opportunity to appraise the breasts of women after they have become mothers—at my gym, in the communal dressing rooms, in the steam room—and I have yet to see any that truly remained unchanged after childbirth. I'm so sorry your Girlfriends had to be the ones to tell you, but it is better that you know it going in. Feel free to live in your disbelieving dreamworld now, but read this part of *The Girlfriends' Guide* again in about a year and then talk to me.

Any woman who tells you that she was small-chested until after she had children and then developed a voluptuous body (such as a certain celebrity we all know) either suffers from an inability to distinguish reality from fantasy or has neglected to mention a critical bit of plastic surgery. The following rule of thumb holds true for just about every woman who has borne children and yet has full and perky breasts that stand at attention without the help of underwire, whether she is a movie star or someone in your yoga class. IF THEY ARE FULL AND ROUNDED AND STAND UP ON THEIR OWN, THEY ARE NOT REAL. If you know any substantiated exceptions to this rule, do us all a favor and keep them to yourself. Anyone who assures you that after nursing your baby, your breasts will return to their pre-pregnancy loveliness either did not have nice breasts to begin with or is a La Leche League recruitment officer. Many women, including several of my Girlfriends, considered not nursing their babies, and this concern about trashing their breasts was one of the reasons why. By the way, *The Girlfriends' Guide* thinks that the breast is best if it suits your temperament and lifestyle (especially if it is given up by the time the baby can unbutton your shirt herself). And one reason we are so cavalier about this, besides our belief that your body is no longer yours for the next year or so anyway, is because we are convinced that most breast-deflating comes from losing the weight after pregnancy, not from nursing.

The Behind

You may ask yourself sometime during this pregnancy, "If the baby is in my belly, why is it my butt that's growing?" After a few visits to the zoo and a lot of Discovery Channel watching, I have developed my own explanation for why our hips and butts get involved in pregnancy when it doesn't really seem to be any of their business. Have you ever noticed how the chimpanzees and orangutans walk around with their babies on the back of their hips? Maybe nature intended to provide a rumble seat for our little ones, since only kangaroos and other marsupials are blessed with those handy pouches to tuck their babies in. If my theory is correct that this fat pocket is a holdover from our caveman days, then a few more evolutionary generations of Bugaboos and Maclarens should eliminate this problem entirely.

Then again, there is the traditional explanation that nature wants to ensure that the fetus won't starve, so it forces your body to carry around emergency food supplies in the form of fat on your hips, butt, upper arms—and let's not forget the face! That might explain the existence of the fat, but it doesn't explain why the butt takes on the roundness of a bubble. Remember this anatomical fact when we get to chapter 10, "Looking the Best You Can," because there is nothing worse than a too short shirt hiking up over that bubble to make you look like the old *Saturday Night Live* family the Wide-Asses. Even if you don't get very fat, your backside will take on a new silhouette.

Hair (and Nails)

One last area of accelerated growth is your hair. It's as if the protein button is permanently pushed ON in pregnancy, since most pregnant women find that their hair seems longer and thicker than ever before. Not only does your hair grow faster than usual, but your body is also signaling your scalp not to release old hairs as frequently as it used to. Therefore you get more *and* longer hair. This is one of nature's consolation prizes: You get big as a punch buggy, but you have more lustrous hair than a shampoo model.

If that was all there were to this hair business, it would be a dream come true—but there always seems to be a catch, doesn't there? The first catch is your scalp, which we will discuss shortly. Another problem is that sometimes it's not just the hair on your head that accelerates in growth, it can be the hair all over your body. Some women find their pubic hair stretching farther up their bellies and down their thighs. Others sprout a hair or two along the outline of their nipples. And some find a downy fuzz growing on their jawline and cheeks or on their backs between their shoulders.

The texture of your hair and its personality will also change during pregnancy. Because of this, another cardinal rule from *The Girlfriends' Guide* is NEVER GET A PERM WHEN YOU ARE PREGNANT! Chances are good that if you do, you will find that only some of your hair "grabs" the perm, and that other huge portions remain straight and unaffected, leaving you looking like Napoleon Dynamite.

A big dilemma for the pregnant woman is whether to continue coloring her hair during pregnancy. As opinionated as *The Girlfriends' Guide* can be, we will control ourselves long enough to present both sides. This is a decision that you must make after consultation with your doctor. Some people would no sooner put chemicals on their hair when pregnant than drink a Red Bull. They wish to protect their unborn children from as many toxic substances as possible; in a world teeming with pollution, malathion, and radon, the last thing they want to do is voluntarily ingest more chemicals.

There. That said, we can get on with other opinions, namely mine. Being an older mother, I was certain that my natural hair color was probably not only boring brown, but boring brown with a couple of grays (YIKES!). I am not sure, because I haven't seen my natural hair color in nearly two decades, but it seems like a reasonable assumption. Therefore, it would take nothing short of a nuclear disaster for me to show the world my real hair. Then again, I was known to drink a Diet Coke now and then, too. So shoot me!

Before you reach for that peroxide bottle, however, you should know a couple of things. First, because your hair will be growing so much faster now, you will need to color your roots more often than before. Unless you color your hair yourself at home, this will soon become expensive. If you are, like Christina Aguilera, a platinum blonde of brunette descent, you could have a stripe down the middle of your head every two to three weeks. Second, the smell of ammonia and bleach will be unbearable early in your pregnancy; after all, they are nearly unbearable when you're not pregnant. And, third, you may just be too plain old tired to get to the beauty salon as often as before. These are all good reasons to change your hair to a shade that is closer to the one God gave you so that you can get away with less frequent coloring, or to consider alternatives to permanent hair color, such as rinses or vegetable dyes.

The last and perhaps most important rule about hair during pregnancy is this: DO NOT CUT YOUR HAIR OFF WHEN YOU ARE PREGNANT! This advice may sound like it's out of left field right now, but trust us, there will come a time when you will consider cutting all your hair off. This is never a good idea, because a very pregnant woman who wants to cut her hair is not really looking for a new hairdo, she is looking for a new, *nonpregnant* look, and I'm afraid that's too tall an order for a haircut. I know how simple and carefree a short, boyish bob can sound at about seven months, but pregnancy is not the time to try it out. Don't forget, your face is pregnant now, too, and you need bone structure to pull off that Natalie Portman look. Sure, Mia Farrow looked adorable with short hair when she was pregnant in *Rosemary's Baby,* but remember, that was a *pretend* pregnancy. And besides, remember *that* baby? Between us, Girlfriends, you may end up looking more like Schlitze the Pinhead than a gamine if you cut your hair when you are ripe with child. And your partner, whose nerves are already pretty raw at this point, will probably snap if you cut your hair, since most men prefer long hair under any circumstances, even if it makes you look like a cross-dresser.

To let you know how overwhelming this haircutting urge can be, I'll relate my own experience. I have always known this prohibition against changing hairstyles in pregnancy, and I was able to withstand the temptation for three whole pregnancies. Then, during my fourth pregnancy, I decided to test the rule. Perhaps I thought it was a stupid rule, or that it didn't apply to me (even though I was the one who made it up). Who knows what insanity was racing through my brain? So in I went and lopped all my hair off, and never did a human head more resemble a coconut. It wasn't a bad haircut. But if you are puffy and overtired, no haircut in the world will make you look better. You will look like a grape on a watermelon even if Oscar Blandi himself styles you.

The other protein in your body that will be growing as fast as your hair will be your fingernails and toenails. If you have previously had the flimsy kind of nails that bend and peel, you will love the new nails you get to enjoy during pregnancy. They are not only growing faster, they are harder and healthier. In fact, if you notice your nails getting worse rather than better at this time, you should discuss it with your doctor immediately, because it could indicate that your body is not getting enough protein to keep you and the baby healthy.

This is a good time to pay more attention to manicures and pedicures. If you can find the time and the money, have them done in a salon. You could use an hour or two of someone massaging your hands and feet. Besides, as pregnancy progresses, only the most limber and determined of us will still be able to cut and paint our own toenails. You will enjoy having pretty hands, expecially when you feel that everything else about your appearance is questionable.

Around the third trimester, you will be tempted to ignore the pedicures, not just because they become impossible to do yourself, but because you so rarely see your own feet anymore that you never notice if they look groomed. But this is when pedicures become particularly important, because your toes are usually right in your obstetrician's face during internal exams, and even more so during the long hours of labor and delivery. I gave up the bikini waxes about seven months into pregnancy, mostly because I couldn't see my pubic hairs from any angle, but I ferociously kept up appearances where my feet were concerned.

One Girlfriend took this advice so much to heart that when her water broke, she immediately ran for the nail polish. She sat on a staircase to paint her toes so that she could reach them all. Then she slipped on some rubber sandals and left for the hospital. By the time she finished checking in and getting to a room, her pedicure was dry. Now, that's a woman with standards!

Your Skin

Pregnancy can be a trying experience for your skin. First there is the obvious challenge of stretching enough to allow for the growth of another human being within your body. You may sometimes wonder, too, whether your skin will be able to encompass your gigantic breasts without suffering some kind of permanent damage. The bottom line, of course, is that the skin will stretch to meet these challenges. Have you ever heard of anyone who just spontaneously explodes under the pressure of pregnancy, even in the *National Enquirer*? But this stretching will not be entirely without incident. Let's talk about some of the specifics, shall we?

Stretch Marks
Stretch marks are lines on your skin that look like runs in your stockings, if you can imagine your breasts, behind, and belly wearing stockings. They occur when the skin stretches more than it wants to. During pregnancy they look rather reddish or purplish, but long after the baby is born they will look almost white or silver. All Girlfriends ask each other if they got stretch marks, as if to determine whether God was fair when he made it happen. It's sort of like "I got them, and I will be pretty disappointed if I'm the only one in our gang who did, damn it!"

Here's the news on stretch marks: THE ONLY SURE WAY TO GUARANTEE THAT YOU WON'T GET STRETCH MARKS IS TO MAKE SURE YOU ARE BORN TO A WOMAN WHO DIDN'T GET THEM, AND WHOSE MOTHER DIDN'T GET THEM EITHER. In other words, it is largely a matter of heredity whether you will get stretch marks. What about all of those lotions and oils that are for sale? you ask. Useless! Go ahead and massage them in if you like the smell or if you believe that it doesn't hurt to cover all the bases, but they cannot fight genetics.

Those creams, lotions, and oils *can* come in handy for another reason. They might help soothe the itchiness that comes from skin being mercilessly stretched. Some women really suffer with this itchiness, and their temptation, especially when they get undressed for the day, is to scratch their belly and sides until their skin bears fingernail marks. If this gets really out of control for you, tell your doctor, because creams and antihistamines can be prescribed to keep you from tearing yourself to shreds. But if you are only mildly itchy, it might be pleasurable to massage yourself with these magic salves. If you can get your mate to play along, you can use the lotions and oils to lubricate all sorts of things!

By the way, I have never really found stretch marks to be the odious things that some people think they are. I suppose if you put on a bikini and go out for a sunbath, they can be a tad imperfect, but artificial tans cover them nicely and everyone now knows that a real suntan is a terrible idea.

Your Complexion

Quite frequently, newly pregnant women get pimples for the first time since they were teenagers. Hormones are potent chemicals, and they can mess up your skin almost as much as they mess up your emotions. Talk to your doctor about whether you can continue with your Proactiv regimen, but giving extra attention to keeping your complexion clean is a must. Trust us—this will pass as soon as your body equalizes its hormonal seesaw. In the meantime, just *don't pick*! Besides, if you take extra time making your hair look great, no one will notice your spots.

Again on the subject of hair, you may find it heavy and dull early in pregnancy. This is because your scalp, being skin, is subject to the same hormonal mayhem that is affecting your face. You may find that your scalp is oily or flaky for the first time in your life. The Girlfriends offer this general rule: Always have scrupulously clean hair when pregnant. If you think you can go one more day before you need to shampoo, you will generally be wrong. Heavy hair that hugs your skull will do absolutely nothing to draw attention away from your face and its problems.

Another way in which your skin might tick you off is by getting little red dots or broken capillaries. They are small and not particularly unattractive, but they may bug you. The red pin-dots usually come during the pregnancy, and the broken capillaries are usually the result of a lot of long, hard pushing during delivery. You may want to have them removed by a doctor after the pregnancy, since they tend to stay with you long after the child has grown up and gone to college.

In keeping with your general condition of overall fertility, you may find strange things growing on your skin. Lots of my Girlfriends got skin tags, which are little teeny flaps of extra skin. Two popular places for a tag are under your arm and on your eyelid. Perhaps this is because there's skin rubbing on skin in these locations. One of my Girlfriends even got one on her labia. They aren't dangerous at all, unless you pick them, in which case they could become infected. Just leave them alone, and later they can easily be removed.

Changing Colors

Pregnancy does an interesting thing to your pigmentation, a subject that is not often discussed by anyone other than your Girlfriends. You will change colors in all sorts of places. The first change you may notice is that your nipples get darker. If they were pink before, they will look more purple when you are pregnant, and if they were beige before, they will turn brown. The nipples and the surrounding pigmented area also get substantially larger, so that what was once the size of a half-dollar may grow to about the size of a small pancake. The Girlfriends have found that after pregnancy, the nipples may return to approximately their former size, but it will be a long time before they regain their former color, if ever.

Here's a news flash that your doctor will probably never point out to you (unless you live in Berkeley): Your labia (the "lips" of your vagina) change color, too, when you are pregnant. They get darker and more engorged with blood. Take a hand mirror and look for yourself if you don't believe me. Just as your nipples get bigger, so do your sexual organs. This change might sound a bit alarming to you at first, but nobody really sees it besides your partner and your doctor, so don't be embarrassed. Of course, you may want to reassure your partner that this is a completely natural state, because oral sex could seem to him like an athletic feat at this time.

The best news about the changes "down below" is that many Girlfriends feel as if they are constantly sexually aroused because their organs are engorged with blood. My Girlfriend Tracy says that she became nearly orgasmic if she walked fast because her legs rubbing together was like never-ending foreplay. Kind of makes a trip to the mall an entirely new experience, don't you think? But one minor drawback to the swelling down there is the sudden inability to aim your urine stream. I know that might sound like a meaningless complaint, but you will often be asked to pee in a specimen cup, and it would be nice if you could do so without getting your hand wet. (Incidentally, my Girlfriend Shannon says that the lips on her face, not just her vaginal lips, also got fuller and darker. Wouldn't you just love to have that happen to you? My lips stayed pretty much the same and I still lived for my lipstick pencil, but who knows, you may be as lucky as Shannon.)

Pigment can also play nasty tricks on pregnant women. Some Caucasian women get what is diabolically described as "the mask of pregnancy" on their face, which usually looks as if you got a skier's tan on your cheeks and forehead, but that you had sunblock on the rest of your face. This irregular coloring goes away after pregnancy, but it can take a while. Stay out of the sun because it only makes matters worse, and try foundation makeup to blend everything together.

Almost every pregnant woman will eventually get a pigment stripe (we call it a *treasure trail* around here) that extends from the top of her pubic hair toward her belly button. We have no explanations for this; we just know it happened to all of us. It was less noticeable on the Girlfriends with more olive or brown in their skin, but on the Irish girls like me, it was pretty obvious. People will tell you that this irregular pigmentation goes away after pregnancy, but it took a couple of years after my last baby was born for mine to disappear. Maybe it's just my imagination, but I think I can still see that trail when I slouch and my baby belly folds over itself. I also think the fine hair that covers my belly has remained darker in the middle. Of course, my belly has not seen the light of day since my first pregnancy, so the contrast between light skin and dark hair is glaringly apparent. No wonder millions of men are fans of Victoria's Secret models. A really good stomach is rarely seen by the father of young children, especially in the privacy of his own bedroom.

4

"I Never Imagined My Body Could Feel Like This!"

PEOPLE TEND TO concentrate on the millions of external physical changes that occur to pregnant women, but the internal changes, not even including those in your uterus, are equally dramatic. As we have pointed out, pregnancy is not limited to your womb, it is a full-body experience, and you may be shocked by how strange and different your body will feel. Everything from stuffy noses to burping can be pregnancy-related.

Your Digestion

A pregnant woman's digestive processes are slowed way down by pregnancy hormones. Evidently, nature wants to ensure that every last vitamin and mineral is extracted from every morsel of food that you eat, so it lets the food sit in your stomach longer than usual. What that means for you can be reduced to two words: *burping* and *farting*.

You may be loath to admit it, but if you take a poll of partners of pregnant women, they will be unanimous in their astonishment at how much free-floating gas there is. All that food just sitting around in your intestines ferments, and you become carbonated. The indelicacy of this condition suggests to me that pregnancy is one of life's best reminders that we are just a few generations removed from dragging our knuckles on the ground when we walk. But if you start thinking that life is unfair, making women endure such a humiliating experience as pregnancy, remember this: It is usually men who go bald.

Let's start with the flatulence. It isn't much of a problem if you spend a lot of time alone or with children under the age of four. In fact, young children are deeply respectful of people who can pass wind on command. It may shock and offend your partner, but even the most fastidious pregnant women soon tire of leaping out of bed or fluffing the sheets surreptitiously, and they soon just let it rip with little regard to whether their beloved mate is present. But, in our inimitable way of caring more about what near-strangers think of us than about what our mates think, being out in public can be fraught with anxiety for those of us with gas. Unfortunately, most of us are not as well-adjusted as my Girlfriend Corki, who will stand up in a small gathering of people and leave the room, announcing over her shoulder, "Excuse me, but I have to fart now." The rest of us feel the slightest intestinal pressure and rush to the ladies' room, praying the whole way that no one else is in there.

Burping is equally hard to control. You can be in the middle of telling an interesting story, and out sneaks a little belch, as if it were an exclamation point. These burps often come out of nowhere with no warning, leaving the burper as shocked as her audience. And pregnant burps are not the short, little gasps that most women insist they make; they are long, ripping sounds that would make any adolescent boy jealous.

Unless your doctor will allow you to take antacids, which we will discuss later in more detail, there really aren't that many things you can do to relieve all this gas. You should probably avoid carbonated drinks and see if that helps. It seems to the Girlfriends, though, that the biggest gas offenders are precisely the foods that you are supposed to eat to make a healthy baby—things like broccoli, spinach, and cauliflower. What's worse, these foods give an aroma to the burps, as well.

Another effect of this relaxation of your digestive muscles can be heartburn. Heartburn, in case you have never had the joy of experiencing it, feels just like it sounds. It is a burning sensation at the base of your esophagus—usually on the left side, it seems—and it can often go hand in hand with burping. It's like an upset stomach, but it's up higher, closer to your chest.

Some women suffer from heartburn throughout their entire pregnancy. Others don't succumb until the baby has grown large enough to put pressure on the muscle, interfering with its closing tightly, that keeps food down in the stomach where it belongs. This can result in stomach acids leaking out. Certain foods seem to make heartburn worse, much like the burping agents, but while I personally was willing to forgo my ration of legumes and brussels sprouts in the name of keeping the burn and gas down, I could not give up my daily ration of peanut M&M's, and they were the worst culprits of all.

If you are lucky, and if you have selected your obstetrician well, you will be allowed to take antacids. Antacids become a pregnant woman's best friend, and it is wise to have them with you at all times. My Girlfriend Julee had huge bottles of the chewable kind in her car, beside her bed, and at work. When you want an antacid, you *really* want one, and you want it *now.* They can be chalky and disgusting, even if they do now come in a rainbow of fruit flavors and promise to dissolve immediately, but, believe me, they actually begin to taste good after a while. A Girlfriends' tip: Always check your mouth in a mirror after eating an antacid because they can leave you with white, chalky stuff on your lips or at the corners of your mouth, making you look as if you are on antipsychotic medication.

One last important bit of information regarding heartburn: No matter what people may try to tell you, HEARTBURN DOES NOT MEAN THAT YOUR BABY WILL BE BORN WITH LOTS OF HAIR. I had heartburn so bad in all four of my pregnancies that I could have spit fire, and all my kids were born as bald as Uncle Fester.

Morning Sickness

As soon as a woman announces that she is pregnant, people ask her if she is feeling sick yet. This is because the stereotypical pregnancy includes a good season of nausea. This nausea, with or without vomiting, is called morning sickness. The Girlfriends and I think that it should be called something more accurate and suitably dramatic, such as "progesterone poisoning." Calling it morning sickness is particularly misleading because it can strike you at *any* time of the day or night. Some women even find that they feel seminauseous all their waking hours.

There is some good news about morning sickness. First, not everyone experiences it. Second, if you do have it, it should go away by the end of the first three months, never to return again (please don't hold me to this). Third, a popular, old-fashioned belief is that the worse your morning sickness, the less likely you are to have a miscarriage. I guess it is believed that the babies of particularly green mothers are already exercising such control over their mothers' systems that nothing is going to get rid of them. All I know is, every time my doctor's nurse asked me how I was feeling and I answered, "Sick," she smiled and replied, "Good!" And fourth, if you feel unbearably wretched soon after learning you're pregnant, you might just have twins in there.

The first and foremost Girlfriends' rule about morning sickness is this: IF YOU GET MORNING SICKNESS, IT DOES NOT MEAN THAT YOU HAVE DONE ANYTHING WRONG DURING YOUR PREGNANCY OR THAT YOU ARE AMBIVALENT ABOUT HAVING THIS BABY! Remember how PMS and cramps used to be considered psychosomatic, and doctors told women that they were only experiencing these manifestations because they were weak or crazy? Then they realized the massive hormonal fluctuations that women experience each month would bring the Wolverine to his knees, if only he had ovaries. Some assholes still suggest that you are barfing your brains out because you are not sure if you are ready to become a mother. Heck, if that were the case, then all women with half a brain would be vomiting all the time, because any fool is smart enough to know that motherhood is a scary business. If you feel nauseous, it's probably because you and progesterone just don't get along. That's it; nothing more.

Morning sickness and seasickness have a lot in common. I have had the nausea that comes with pregnancy, and I have been on a round-bottomed boat in a storm at sea, and the experiences were really quite similar. For example, they both strike an otherwise healthy person. They also have what I call a "head component"; your equilibrium is affected and you might feel dizzy or spacey. I found no relief from seasickness or morning sickness in throwing up, as there can be with stomach flu or food poisoning. Some of my Girlfriends felt otherwise about this, but my experience was that I barfed, I continued to feel sick, and I barfed some more. For this reason, it doesn't really pay to stick your finger down your throat in a desperate attempt to rid your body of the offending poison, since it isn't in your stomach.

Since "progesterone poisoning" has little to do with what you have eaten, you don't stop vomiting simply because you don't have any more food in your stomach. You just move on to the dry heaves or, worse, spitting up stomach bile. Yet even though most women do not get sick *because* of something they have eaten, the sight or smell of particular foods can accelerate the gagging. That, too, is true of seasickness. A whiff of cottage cheese can send a victim of either malady running for the toilet, or the side of the ship, even if she hasn't actually eaten any of it.

You may be asking yourself right now, "How do I know if I will have morning sickness in my pregnancy?" The answer is "You can't predict." Even if you have been pregnant before and sailed right past morning sickness, it doesn't mean you won't get it this time or some other time. Some of my Girlfriends suggest that there is a link between the gender of the baby and whether you will be nauseous. They seem to feel that carrying a girl might make you sicker than carrying a boy. I have no idea if this is true, and I was ill with all four of my kids, so it sounds a little like hoodoo to me. I would imagine that the "scientific" explanation could be the presence of the extra female hormones that a baby girl might share with your body—a sort of estrogen overload. But for every Girlfriend who has told me that she was sicker with her girl babies, I have another who swears that pregnancies with boys were more nauseating. Some studies have indicated that we women recognize boy fetuses as *foreign*, what with their Y chromosome and testosterone, and that could make us sick. By the way, another old wives' tale is that baby girls make your face distort more, and I *swear* that was true with me, but that's getting off on another tangent.

Morning sickness is not necessarily one of the first physical signs that tell you that you are pregnant. What usually happens is, you find out you are pregnant and you feel pretty normal in the digestive sense for another couple of weeks. You will be tempted to start congratulating yourself that your superior health and positive attitude (or the power of prayer) have spared you the nausea that lesser mortals have to endure. Then one morning you walk downstairs in your nightie to get some orange juice from the refrigerator. You open the door of the fridge and get a whiff of last night's meat loaf, and next thing you know, you are puking in the kitchen sink.

Morning sickness does not strike all its victims with equal intensity. Its severity can almost be measured on a sliding scale. At one end are those lucky ones who have one green moment and then never feel a bit of nausea for the rest of their pregnancy. At the other end are those who vomit so much that their doctors put them in the hospital for intravenous fluids and, occasionally, medication to stop the incessant sickness. This is a condition called *hyperemesis,* and it is miserable for the mommy and potentially dehydrating and exhausting to her and her baby.

Before I knew how awful the condition could be, I actually felt a pang of envy for those women who were on the nausea diet, even if it meant that they vomited frequently, because I was getting fatter by the day. Isn't that so sick? I'm ashamed, but I share it with you because we're Girlfriends. Over time, I learned that even those pregnant women who were sick as dogs in the first trimester ended up gaining as much weight as we who never met a meal we couldn't force down. It pays to be careful about what your obsessive mind wishes for because you could end up gaining sixty-five pounds and hurling between every bite.

I have one Girlfriend, Mary, who was so used to having constant nausea with all three of her pregnancies that she just decided to go on with her life as if nothing were unusual. She would go about her daily business, stopping to vomit when it became necessary, then resume the task at hand. She didn't go anywhere without knowing in advance where the nearest bathroom was, so that she could streak to it should the need arise. (BTW, I have recently seen commercials for overactive-bladder medications that give away Frommer's guides to toilets around the world, so you might want to go to their website and ask for one.) Mary also kept towels on the passenger seat of her car so that she wouldn't vomit all over herself when she was caught in a traffic jam. I was always so impressed with her matter-of-factness when I saw her at Mommy and Me classes with two kids and pregnant with a third. She would calmly, but quickly, excuse herself from a verse or two of "The Wheels on the Bus Go Round and Round," go vomit, rinse, and come back to the group in time for the part about the wipers on the bus going swish, swish, swish. We all knew where she had been and what she had done, but she never mentioned it, let alone complained about it. She became a hero to the rest of us, who were complaining about everything all the time.

In the middle of the spectrum is where you will find most of us. We have our good days and our days when we want to die. On the bad days, even staying in bed doesn't provide relief, because we feel just as horrid lying down as we do standing up. So we generally get up and face the day, just counting the hours till we can go to sleep and start a new—and, we pray, better—day. For those of us in the middle, morning sickness doesn't necessarily mean constant vomiting. In fact, I only vomited a few times with each pregnancy, but I felt mildly ill much of the time. It wasn't unusual for me to have to leave meetings or luncheons to get some fresh air during the first trimester of my pregnancies because I was afraid of either fainting or gagging in front of people I didn't think would understand. I wish that I could tell you a secret remedy that would make all pregnancy-related nausea disappear, but I haven't found it in years of looking. What follows, however, is a list of my Girlfriends' guidelines:

The 10 Commandments of Morning Sickness

1. Eat Small Amounts of Bland Foods All Day Long.

2. Don't Eat Anything That Doesn't Smell Appealing to You.

3. Eat Something at Around 4:00 a.m., or After Your Last Middle-of-the-Night Visit to the Toilet.

4. Take Your Prenatal Vitamins at Night, or Stop Altogether Until You Are Feeling Better. (Your Doctor May Want You to Take Folic Acid Supplements in the Meantime.)

5. Do Not Take Your Vitamins with Citrus Juice.

6. When Nothing Sounds Appetizing, Try a Bowl of Cereal with Milk or a Piece of Sweet Fruit.

7. If the Thought of Chewing Any Kind of Food Makes You Sick, Try Sucking on Natural Licorice Drops (They Can Be Soothing).

8. Try Wearing the Elastic Wristbands That Are Sold in Pharmacies to Prevent Seasickness.

9. Skip the Saltines Unless You Have a Real Craving for Them (Which I Can't Imagine, Unless You Are a Parrot).

10. Follow Your Cravings. If You Really Want Some Particular Type of Food, There Is a Good Chance It Will Actually Make You Feel a Little Better. (Just Be Careful If Your Cravings Are Consistently for Oreos and DoveBars, as Mine Were.)

Most women find that morning sickness disappears at right about the three-month mark. It is truly a magical feeling the day you wake up, brush your teeth without activating your gag reflex, get dressed without having to pause to put your head in the toilet, and go to the kitchen eagerly thinking of breakfast. And it happens just like that: One day you are miserable and cooling your cheeks on the bathroom floor, and the next day you've never felt better.

Your Bowels

As I have said before, there is really no aspect of your physical being that is unaffected by pregnancy, and this even applies to your bowel movements. First of all, if you are taking one of the popular brands of prescription prenatal vitamins, you may find that your poops are the color of tire rubber. I think it has something to do with all the iron you are taking, but it's just one more thing about your life that will seem strange.

And, as if you don't feel full enough down there already, with the baby and the fluid and the placenta and God knows what else all jammed into an area that you once were proud to show off in a crop top, pregnancy adds one more ingredient: constipation. Yes, you may notice that you just aren't the same "regular" gal you were before you were pregnant. Perhaps it is the iron in your prenatal vitamins, again, or it may just be the relaxation of your entire digestive tract, but this can be a real annoyance for pregnant women.

How upsetting you will find this unpredictability of bowel movements will depend on a variety of factors. My Girlfriend Andrea determines the mood of her entire day based on a successful BM in the morning, whether she is pregnant or not. Constipation can also be particularly upsetting if you're already uncomfortable about how round your stomach is becoming. And if you're begining to feel more than a little pissed off at how unfamiliar your body is in so many ways, this can be the straw that breaks the camel's back.

Constipation is one area where I remained fairly relaxed, probably because I had never heard of anyone succumbing to a poop explosion, and because anal issues are generally not where my neuroses lie. What goes in must eventually come out, no matter how hard and dark, is my philosophy. Many of my Girlfriends disagree, however, and they were willing to try anything short of scheduling colonics to rid themselves of that "full of shit" feeling.

Traditional books on pregnancy will tell you to increase the amount of fiber you eat and to drink more water. I believe, however, that you can eat bran and drink water until you're ready to explode and your bowel movements will not really get any more manageable. I think that ingesting something more akin to WD-40 and dynamite would be much more effective (but not particularly well-tolerated by the baby).

Talk to your doctor if you are constipated. Don't be ashamed to have such an indelicate conversation with him or her; believe me, far more indelicate things are going to happen in your relationship in the near future. Ask if you can take fiber tablets such as psyllium husks, or a fiber drink. If things get really stopped up, ask about taking a stool softener. I took Colace, a small, gelatinous pill, and it really got things moving after three or four days of use (plus it was a cinch to swallow, which is much appreciated on those gagging days).

JUST MAKE SURE THAT WHATEVER YOU TAKE CONTAINS NO LAXATIVES. Laxatives can really screw up your digestion, you can get "addicted" to them, and they can make your stomach cramp up as in labor. Not to mention that the last thing your little baby needs is something to make *her* poop uncontrollably.

My Girlfriend Denise reminded me of one of the most disconcerting aspects of pregnancy "elimination": the public restroom. Sometimes pregnant women find they must work hard to accomplish a bowel movement. In fact, some of my Girlfriends have said that they remember times they pushed so hard to "move" that they got sweaty at their hairline and made humiliating grunting noises. This can be horrifying enough in the privacy of your own home, but it is much, much worse if you are at work and using the employees' bathroom. It isn't so bad in a very public place like Disney World or the beach because, honestly, what do you care what complete strangers think? (Unless, of course, they tap on the door to see if you are all right, or worse, shout from their place in the line forming outside your door, asking if you plan to spend the day in there.) But to have the office gossip or your own secretary in the stall next to you can be so inhibiting that you would rather succumb to fecal poisoning than do what it takes to poop.

The bright side to this difficulty in pooping is that you can consider those big-effort eliminations to be practice runs for delivery—because a proper delivery push feels *exactly* like the most difficult bowel movement you have ever had in your life. Keep this sensation in mind, and you will know what to do when the doctor tells you it is time to push.

This description of forcing a movement may run afoul of everything your good, overly attentive mother has told you since you stopped wearing diapers. Remember, she said, "Don't push too hard or you'll get hemorrhoids." And guess what? This time Mother may have known what she was talking about. Nonetheless, pushing too hard sometimes happens without our realizing it until it is too late, which leads us nicely to:

Hemorrhoids

If you are like me, you have grown up seeing "those" commercials, but you never really paused to think about *where* those people were putting that miraculous cream or wiping those little pads—or *why* they were doing it in the first place. Well, my innocent little Girlfriend, they were putting it around their anuses, and they were stooping to that indignity because they had little protrusions like peas down there that hurt and itched them to distraction. Don't you just want to scream? It is almost too horrifying to talk about, but as your Girlfriend, I will.

There are various ways to get hemorrhoids, so it is rather like running an obstacle course: You may successfully have leapt over the fence, but you may still fall into the mud pit. First, you can get hemorrhoids (which colorful older folks call piles, for reasons I don't even want to speculate about) from pushing too hard to move your bowels. We have just discussed this, so you know that I am not blaming you. Too much pressure down there can cause some of the anal tissue to herniate and stick out, either individually or in little clusters like grapes.

Another way you can get them is just by virtue of being pregnant, hard poops or not. You see, the weight of the baby and all the other stuff in your abdomen that is supporting it gets so heavy that it can cut off the circulation in the veins and arteries down there, much as a car tire rolling over a garden hose will stop water from coming out. When the rosy area down there gets its blood all pooled up, it's grape time again.

Then, just when you think that you have dodged all the hemorrhoid bullets that nature can shoot your way, it's DELIVERY TIME! That was it for me—my Armageddon, my Alamo, my Little Bighorn. I was just fine, black poops and all, until I pushed my first baby, and evidently, part of my rectum out. After the epidural wore off, I hurt in that general area, but I had had an episiotomy and a small tear that required some stitches, so I attributed the pain to those and didn't do any investigating for the first couple of days. Besides, I was not particularly eager to touch any stitches down there, anyway.

When I got home from the hospital and took a shower, I absentmindedly soaped up to wash my "privates," and I nearly fainted dead away with the shock of what I felt. In the soft tissue around my anus were these firm, rounded clumps of tissue. It felt as though my insides were on the outside.

I immediately went to bed and cried. (At least until a certain newcomer started wailing even louder.) I had no idea what I had felt, but I was certain that no one else had ever experienced anything like it before, and that I would probably die of it (or at least require a rectum tuck). I was so mortified that I didn't mention my condition to anyone—not my husband (who doesn't have the stomach for such things, anyway), not my Girlfriends (who would, I was afraid, pity me and know that I was disfigured), and *certainly* not my doctor, who would tell me it was cancer.

Finally, after not having heard from me since the delivery, my doctor called to see how I was doing, and I blurted out, "There is something growing out of my behind and it hurts worse than my stitches!" I was shocked and relieved to learn that he knew exactly what I was talking about, and that he even had some suggestions to make me feel better. I couldn't believe it—there were actually prescription creams to shrink the hemorrhoids and to lessen the pain and irritation. My doctor also prescribed suppositories, which I suppose were intended to do the same shrinking and relieving on my insides or to ease me back into pooping.

But I can't tell you if they worked because, five years later, they are still in my medicine cabinet, unopened. My doctor was crazy if he thought I was going to try to shove something up there in my condition.

My Girlfriend Jaye had such a bad hemorrhoid problem after the birth of her first child that she saw a proctologist during her second and third pregnancies. Evidently he gave her cortisone shots in her you-know-what. While the thought of that procedure makes me go numb, Jaye assures me that they didn't really hurt and that they saved her from a shower horror like mine. (She giggles when she describes sitting in the proctologist's office, since everyone else in the waiting room was concerned about his prostate and/or was over age seventy. Everyone had a pretty good idea of what part of her anatomy was being treated because, let's face it, no one goes to a proctologist for a second opinion about open-heart surgery.)

Here is a Girlfriend's list of things to try for relief of hemorrhoids (subject, of course, to your doctor's approval):

- Ask for a prescription cream or ointment to help shrink the hemorrhoids and relieve the discomfort.
- Use witch hazel on cotton pads or use medicated hemorrhoid pads whenever the opportunity arises, and certainly every time you use the toilet. They come ready to throw into your purse or diaper bag and will keep the area clean, temporarily pain-free, and might even help shrink the little buggers.
- Take lots of baths. The warm water is not only soothing (and the weightlessness of your body a relief), but it keeps the area scrupulously clean, which helps prevent infection. Someone may suggest that you take a *sitz bath*. What they are referring to is sitting in a few inches of the hottest water you can stand for twenty to thirty minutes at a time. My personal feeling is that if you have that kind of time on your hands, go to sleep instead. You will forget all about your hemorrhoids while in slumberland.
- Have some kind person go to a pharmacy and buy you a hemorrhoid pillow, which looks like a large, firm doughnut. In fact, if you live in a two-story house, have the kind person buy you two so that, when the baby comes and your pooper is feeling its worst, you don't have to carry both your baby and your doughnut up and down the stairs at the same time.

- Better still, invest in one of those circular baby pillows, bops, which you can find in many mail-order catalogs. You know the ones: They are covered in bright and cheerful cotton, and the baby is supposed to sit in the hole in the middle and be propped up by the surrounding pillow. I have never birthed a baby who wanted to be seated in one of these contraptions, but they sure were great for me.
- Ask your obstetrician to refer you to a proctologist as Jaye's did. Those cortisone shots don't sound half-bad when your insides seem to be spilling out your behind.
- If all else fails, there is always surgery for this area, which you can get after the baby is born. It's even covered by most insurance policies.

5

Pregnancy Insanity

THE PHYSICAL CHANGES brought on by pregnancy are numerous and extreme enough to give a woman whiplash, but they would ultimately be manageable if they weren't accompanied by some pretty hefty emotional changes. The inner life of many pregnant women is scary enough to make their mates anxious and vigilant and their friends impatient and annoyed. I was so bitchy during one of my pregnancies that my friends finally stopped trying to spare my feelings and just told me to "shut up" whenever they had heard enough. Some pregnant women become short-fused and extremely rigid. For example, if we asked my Girlfriend Janis out for lunch, she would have all sorts of rules, such as we had to eat at 12:15 exactly, no sooner and no later, and the restaurant chairs had to have arms or she wouldn't be comfortable enough to digest her food, and that her chair had to have padding or her peepee would ache.

Keep this Girlfriend Rule of Thumb in mind as you read this chapter: CRAZY PEOPLE ARE OFTEN THE LAST TO KNOW THEY ARE CRAZY. Therefore, if you are tempted to skip to the next chapter because you don't see how this one applies to you, think again; you may be crazier than you look (at least to yourself). In fact, ask around, because you may be surprised to learn that you, too, are a victim of Gestational Psychosis. (I made that condition up, so don't go looking for it online.)

One aspect of Pregnancy Insanity feels quite like PMS. The answer to the question "How long will this feeling last?" is "About forty weeks." Like everything else in pregnancy, its severity varies not just from person to person, but from day to day. This will be good news to those of you really feeling the effects of the Insanity, and not-so-good news for those of you who maintain that you have never felt better in your life.

Here is another bit of Girlfriend advice: If your friends who have been pregnant tell you that it was the most emotionally fulfilling and happiest time of their life, don't believe them. Those kinds of comments invariably make you feel that something is wrong with you if you don't feel equally ecstatic, and they are undoubtedly inaccurate. Some strange biological force gives women amnesia about pregnancy, so that they forget the less savory details and see the whole thing in a sort of rosy glow. This is just nature's way of making sure that women get pregnant more than once; if you remembered too much, you might never voluntarily repeat the experience.

What follows are various manifestations of Pregnancy Insanity. You will probably know them all at some time during gestation; let's hope you won't feel them all at the same time!

"I Can't Concentrate Anymore!"

At no time prior to Alzheimer's will you experience such forgetfulness and lack of logical thinking. Part of this feeblemindedness can be attributed simply to the overloading of the pregnant woman's brain circuitry: There is just so damn much to think about. You have to decide who your doctor will be, what hospital you want to deliver the baby in, whether you want to know the baby's gender in advance, whether you should get prenatal genetics testing, how to tell your boss you'll be needing a maternity leave, how to tell your mate that your mother will be staying with you for a few weeks after the baby comes, and so on and so on. It is only rational and natural that you should feel confused and out of control at a time like this.

But there is more to this aspect of Pregnancy Insanity. Many pregnant women also exhibit a sort of foggy, daydreamy behavior. You know what I am talking about: the state of mind that allows you to drive all the way home from work with your dry cleaning on the roof of your car, or to sit in a meeting for hours and not recall a single point that was made.

Perhaps you and your baby are already talking to each other: planning, imagining one another's face, being shy about your first meeting. Perhaps you are wondering what a son will be like, or whether your daughter will be nicer to you as a teenager than you were to your mother. You wonder if your child will ever do anything to make you burst with pride, as George W. did for Barbara. You worry that the child may do something to totally embarrass you, like George W. did to Barbara. These reveries are so compelling that other people's chatter may seem irrelevant, and you may want to shake them by the shoulders and shout, "Hey, I'm gestating here!"

You might become a bit worried about how this lack of concentration will affect your ability to care for your baby when it is born. Don't fret yet; this absentmindedness is small potatoes compared with how distracted you will be once you have a child in your arms, whom you will worry about until the day you die. Enjoy how low the stakes still are now, because once the baby is born, you will have to worry about more realistic catastrophes, such as setting the baby down someplace and driving off without it.

"Diaper Commercials Make Me Weep!"

One of the more harmless aspects of the emotional spin cycle of pregnancy is how sentimental Girlfriends become. Nearly every mother has a recollection of crying at a diaper or formula commercial on television when she was pregnant. I used to love the commercials for health-care plans that showed babies being born to deliriously happy couples. One night, toward the end of my first pregnancy, I sat in my son's waiting nursery and played a cassette of lullabies and sobbed until my husband worried that I might need to seek professional care.

My Girlfriend Maryann, who recently found out she is pregnant, tells me that she is frequently overwhelmed by her affection for her parents and her husband. She can sob buckets simply by imagining that one of her loved ones might get hit by a truck or struck by lightning before the baby is born. It's as if she is dealing with how vulnerable she feels over the fragility of all life, particularly the lives of those she loves most.

An emotional crisis can occur if you are pregnant during a publicized catastrophe involving a baby. Years ago, when the little girl from Texas called Baby Jessica fell down a hole in her backyard, my Girlfriend Amy got so upset that she was a mess for days. She felt such empathy for the parents that she was unable to eat, sleep, or even talk on the telephone until the child was rescued. Those television news segments on starving children in third world countries are so psychically painful for pregnant women that they often react as if they have sustained a personal loss. Even the pictures of missing children on milk cartons seem like a special call to action for all pregnant women.

The amusing part of this sentimentality is the kinship you immediately feel for all mothers of the world, from Carol Brady to the woman yelling at her whining child at Toys R Us. The world becomes divided into two groups: those who have children and those who do not. And you will be most interested in the subgroup of *women who are pregnant when you are.* When you are pregnant, it seems as though the entire childbearing population is pregnant, too. You can't swing a loaf of bread in a supermarket without hitting a pregnant woman. You check each other out with uncontainable curiosity but with the friendliness of comrades. You try to guess how pregnant your new comrade is (and whether she is looking as good or as bad as you are at this point), and you will have no qualms about asking this complete stranger her entire gestational history.

If you are pregnant at the same time as a celebrity, you will develop a familiarity with her pregnancy that will make you feel "related" to her in some way. For example, you may be pregnant with Gwen Stefani, Reese Witherspoon, one of the president's daughters, or maybe Kate Bosworth or Sienna Miller, and Britney's probably game for a few more—and you'll feel maternal about their children, even though you don't know them. (Though I can't help but feel I know Sean Preston.) Years ago, I saw on the 11:00 p.m. news that the star of a big television series suffered a miscarriage late in her pregnancy. I had my husband wake up immediately and take me to the hospital to make sure that our baby was still safe and alive in my stomach. I swear.

Later, after you have all had your babies, you will keep an eye on these women to see how they are doing getting back into shape. Many of my Girlfriends were traumatized that Kelly Ripa got so thin after her last big fat pregnancy. I myself confess to taking a dark joy when tabloid magazines show unflattering photos of brand-new celebrity mothers caught off guard getting off an airplane after a seven-hour flight with a new baby.

"I Want It and I Want It now!"

Immediate gratification is the goal of most pregnant women. It may appear to the unenlightened that pregnant women are just whimsically indulging themselves and taking advantage of their condition. This is not entirely true. Certain sensations take on a ferocity when you are pregnant that they never had in your nonpregnant state. And God help the person who stands between you and your satisfaction.

For example, a nonpregnant woman can find herself needing to peepee when driving in a car with her mate. When this happens, she might calmly mention to him that she wouldn't mind stopping at the nearest clean bathroom if they should happen to pass one. And she'll probably add that if they don't happen to pass one, she can hold it until they reach their destination.

The scenario changes when the woman is pregnant. Her voice takes on a twinge of hysteria as she blurts out that she has to go to the bathroom. She immediately sounds so desperate that you would swear she is so full that her eyeballs have started to float. Her frightened partner begins to look for an appropriate stop. The next thing he knows, her hand is on the door handle and she is preparing to hurl herself out of the moving car. She has to relieve herself so badly that she is willing to do it anywhere but the front seat of the car. She would consider doing it there, too, but then she would have to sit in it for the rest of the trip. The guy's inability to completely comprehend the urgency of his darling's request to stop can be ground zero for a good hormonal fight, so our best advice to the nonpregnant parties in this situation is this: Don't Ask Questions. Immediately Pull Over and Run Around to Your Mate's Side of the Car. Help Her Out and into a Hiding Place Behind a Tree or Road Sign. And Watch Out for Your Shoes. Remember, Extreme Times Call for Extreme Measures!

If that sort of display regarding urinating shocks your baby daddy, just wait until he sees the Pregnant You when you discover that you are hungry and you have no food within your immediate reach! A pregnant woman's hunger is no moderate or simple hankering. It is a hunger so ferocious that if the car isn't parked in front of some food-selling source within thirty seconds, the hapless man will find himself face-to-face with a sobbing woman who is tearing through the glove compartment trying to find the peppermint candy she picked up at the car wash a month ago.

Perhaps there is some medical explanation, such as a rapid drop in blood-sugar levels or something. I do know that it makes you feel anxious, cranky, and desperate. That is why we Girlfriends suggest that you plan ahead for these hunger crises by keeping food in your car, in your relatives' cars, in your purse, in your office, in your locker, beside your bed . . . well, you get our drift. By the way, mark any food stashed at work with the words *Pregnant Woman's Food—Touch on Pain of Death,* because there is nothing worse than reaching for your last snack only to find that the HR guy ate it. Bags of nuts and grains, granola bars, and bananas are great rations, and they will keep you from streaking into a fast-food drive-

...zy. Thirst, too, is immediate and gripping for a pregnant
...until you try nursing if you want to know what *dying of*
...). So, in addition to the snacks, you should have several
...water strategically placed.

"I Think I Hate My Baby's Father!"

Let's start with the simple premise that, by virtue of being a nonfemale, your partner will have absolutely no idea what it feels like to be you right now. He will not know your anxiety, your ambivalence, your insecurities, or your near-toxic hormonal state. That's enough right there to qualify him for the title of Most Clueless Human. Trust your Girlfriends when we tell you that even if he denies it to your face, your true love thinks that pregnancy has made you irrational, emotional, and unpredictable—all of the things most guys hate in a person, especially the one bearing his off-spring, thereby binding him to her forever. I have found in my interviewing that when wives are present, the new daddies regale me with stories of their brave and pioneering partners who selflessly gave themselves over to pain and deprivation to produce their precious angel babies.

Get these men in a group without the women, however, and the stories of Pregnancy Insanity grow like the legend of The Gerbil. Gary remembers the time his wife lay down on the floor of the frozen-yogurt store because she felt nauseous. He recalls with agonizing embarrassment how the other shoppers had to step over and around her to get to the counter. Then there is Michael, who describes the quantities of food his pregnant wife ate as if she were a human garbage disposal. He goes on to piteously explain how he was never allowed to finish his own meal because his voracious wife attacked his plate with a shovel. All of these husbands roll their eyes and nod in unison when one mentions the impossibility of coming up with the correct answer to the pregnant woman's favorite question: "Do you still love me even though I'm fat?" This one throws them all, because they don't really know whether they are supposed to tell their wives that they would love them no matter what—since that implies that they do, indeed, think their wives are fat—or if it is wiser to say no, they only like thin women, like her.

Few things are more irritating than losing your mind and having someone point that out to you at the same time. Get prepared for comments from your mate like "Aren't you overreacting, just a little?" or "Is this the real you or the pregnant you talking?" How about "You used to be a lot more fun before you got pregnant" or "My chiropractor's wife didn't need any medication when she delivered their baby, and I don't think you should take any either" or "I know you have the flu, but do you really need that antihistamine?"

The chief complaint among the Girlfriends seems to be that our fellas don't find this pregnancy business as overwhelmingly important as we do. They can think of other things for hours, even days on end, while a pregnant woman (especially if it is her first pregnancy) can think of nothing else. To a pregnant woman, even war in the Middle East becomes about her baby in some way: Maybe we pull out of Iraq and there's an oil shortage and she won't have enough gas to get to the hospital when she goes into labor. Men, on the other hand, tend to look at pregnancy as something that possesses their womenfolk but is largely a nonevent until the baby is actually born.

I once called my husband, who was in New York on business, to complain that he clearly did not want the new baby as much as I did. When he rationally asked what evidence I had for this presumption, I told him that, even though I had been pregnant for seven months, he had not spent one single minute thinking about what we were going to name the baby. I'd thought about the baby's name at least twice a day from the day I'd found out I was pregnant, and more often than that after the doctor had told me I was going to have a little girl. My husband seemed to work on the assumption that names were handed out at the hospital.

One way that many husbands can and do share the pregnancy with their wives is by matching them pound for pound in weight gain. So many of my Girlfriends report that their partner put on ten to twenty pounds when they were pregnant. I think I read somewhere that Matt Damon did that very thing. Who knows—maybe they are eating from nervous stress, or maybe they are just keeping their lady company at the feed bin. Some of them actually get cravings along with their mate. I don't think this is really a grand display of empathy, but rather a case of "If you get something, I want it, too"—as in "If you are going to have a banana split, I deserve to have one, too." My husband took this "me, too" business a bit further when he insisted that he caught every malady I had, only he had it worse. If I took to bed with bronchitis, he was sure that he had pneumonia. This is a clever ruse, because no one would ever expect a man with *pneumonia* to take care of a chubby, crazy woman with a little bit of a cough.

What can really be infuriating to a pregnant woman who feels that she is enduring her pregnancy with little or no genuine support or understanding from her partner is the gnawing thought at the back of her mind "It's all his fault. He *did* this to me in the first place." He comes away from a roll in the hay with a satisfied glow and the promise of a good night's sleep, and her life is changed forever. At no time is this blame felt more than during labor and delivery. It's infuriating to be lying in a hospital bed with your uterus contracting like a bucking bronco and seeing your "birth coach" eating something from the cafeteria and watching *Wheel of Fortune.* Life's just not fair sometimes.

"I'm Scared to Death!"

Fear is a common denominator among all pregnant women. It is neck-snapping, the speed with which you can go from feeling joyous to feeling terrified upon learning that you are going to have a baby. First, there is a general sense of alarm at the whole prospect of growing a baby inside you and being responsible for it until the day you die. This is when you might start looking for an escape. Shortly after this, the fears become more specific. You don't just feel a huge, undifferentiated sense of worry, but you can list the individual things that terrify you from moment to moment. The fears usually break down in the following manner:

Fear of Miscarriage

Once you have come to terms with the shock and excitement of learning that you are pregnant, you will discover that sustaining that pregnancy becomes the single most important goal of your life. This fear of losing a pregnancy is not completely irrational. Statistics say that something like one out of five diagnosed pregnancies does end in miscarriage, and the odds vary according to such factors as how old you are, if you are pregnant with multiples, or if you have a history of miscarriage. And if you have ever endured a miscarriage or had a close friend go through one, you know that it is far more than a particularly painful menstrual period. To a woman who is eagerly awaiting the birth of her child, the loss of that child, no matter how early on it is, is cause for great grief and mourning.

For some women, especially those who conceived without much trouble and who have never experienced any threat to a pregnancy, such as bleeding or actual miscarriage, sustaining their pregnancy means little more than using the elliptical machine instead of road racing. For other women, like myself, who tried for years to get pregnant or who for some other reason think that their pregnancy is more fragile, the first three months are characterized by far more precautions.

Almost every pregnancy book on the market will tell you that there is absolutely no reason for a woman with what is known as a "low risk" pregnancy (ask your doctor to classify yours) to curtail her fitness activities in any way. Intellectually, I can begrudgingly accept this wisdom, but emotionally, especially for the precarious first three months, I reject it wholeheartedly. I know that the vast majority of miscarriages that occur in the first trimester are the result of a genetic malformation of the embryo, but I just cannot understand why anyone would want there to be one scintilla of a chance that her taking that ninety-minute kick-boxing class was partly to blame. If you can take it easy, why not do so?

The only reason why not is to live up to some current notion of being a superhuman who can gestate and swing from a trapeze at the same time. Sure, we have all heard of women who have done just that, but what do they have to do with you and your baby? The most important rule of pregnancy is THIS IS NOT A CONTEST! YOU JUST DO WHAT YOU CAN TO SURVIVE THE NINE (TEN) MONTHS AND HAVE A HEALTHY BABY.

I have already told you how many times I turned white as a sheet and ran to the bathroom in dread of seeing blood in my underwear. And I actually did bleed in all four of my pregnancies, and it was terrifying every single time. I took the bleeding episodes as messages from God to go right to bed. I had a new respect for how fragile all life can be. That is why the Girlfriends advise that you cut yourself some slack when you find out you are pregnant. Miscarriages, tragically, do happen, but there is absolutely no reason for you to wonder whether there was anything you could have done to help save the pregnancy, such as give up the cigarettes or the bench-pressing.

Another biological reason that some women worry about miscarriage is a cramping sensation that often occurs in the early part of pregnancy. This cramping feels just like menstrual cramps, and if you feel them in the early weeks, you will swear that this pregnancy business was all a dream and that your period is starting within minutes. I must have been ten weeks pregnant before I stopped sticking sanitary napkins onto my underwear every day, just in case those cramps meant business. If you are feeling them, relax—they almost always mean nothing. If they are painful and accompanied by any bleeding, ignore everything I have just said and contact your doctor.

Fear of Something Being Wrong with Your Baby

Your sometimes uncontrollable fear that your child may be born less than perfect is your first inkling of how vulnerable you will be regarding the well-being of your baby. From now until the day you die (or gratefully succumb to senility), you will fret over the condition of your child. If your baby is not happy and well, neither are you. Here it is, not even born yet, and already you are suffering from the sense of dread about how you will cope if something happens to your child.

We all know that, unfortunately, babies are sometimes born with health problems, just as we all know that older children sometimes get sick or break their bones, need emergency appendectomies, or, God forbid, have even worse things happen. But our fears almost always exceed the probabilities of these things ever occurring. The vast majority of children are born with ten fingers and ten toes, and they manage to survive childhood disasters so successfully that the greatest threat to their well-being is the very real chance that we will kill them ourselves when they are teenagers.

Even with all this in mind, it is impossible to stop rerunning the brain tape that plays out what you will do if something is less than perfect with your baby. This is because you are certain that if something happens to your child, you will have no other option but to die yourself. This kind of intense love and identification with your baby surprises every woman when she first recognizes it. When you comprehend its power, you will begin to understand why you will want to smack a two-year-old who throws sand in your child's eyes or torch a schoolteacher who suggests that your child might not be ready for first grade after all.

Anyway, back to the irrational fears that something will be wrong with your baby. I think that one of the reasons we play out every disastrous scenario in our minds during pregnancy is to toughen our psyches in the event such a horrible thing happens. It's as if we think that if we have imagined it already, the shock or sadness might not be as great as it would be if we were caught blissfully unaware. I don't need to tell you that this is hoodoo thinking at its finest; you know it, too, but it is something most of us need to do.

Many women choose to have various tests to eliminate some of the worries about birth defects. Many states require that mothers give a blood sample for what is known as an alpha-fetoprotein test, which checks for spina bifida and can indicate whether the fetus has a statistically higher chance of being born with Down syndrome. There is also a blood-screening test with genetic markers for Down syndrome.

Ultrasound, which many pregnant women get at least a couple of times during pregnancy, can also reassure you that your child has a heart with all four chambers, a brain, and all the arms and legs it is supposed to have. If the baby is feeling particularly brazen on the day of your ultrasound (or sonogram), you may even see its sex organs and know with reasonable certainty if you are having a boy or girl.

If you are thirty-five or older, you will probably have a genetic test that samples some of the pregnancy matter or the amniotic fluid. These tests are called CVS (chorionic villus sampling) and amniocentesis, respectively. (They will be discussed further in the "Prenatal Tests" chapter.) A good result on these tests eliminates the possibilities of your baby being born with a number of birth defects.

But if you think the worry stops there, you are pitifully mistaken. As soon as you think that your baby is spared the traumas of Tay-Sachs disease or Down syndrome, you creatively come up with other things to obsess about, such as whether it is going to have crossed eyes or ears like Prince Charles's. Worry seems to be a necessary exercise for pregnant women, and for every bit of reassurance you get, you will substitute one more thing to worry about.

Guilt provides all sorts of material for uncontrollable worrying in a pregnant woman. We become convinced that now is the time to pay the piper for all of the terrible things we did to ourselves in our carefree youth. If you, unlike most declared political candidates, actually inhaled when you smoked weed, you will feel faint at the prospect that your chromosomes are forever altered and your baby will have twelve toes. Imagine those of us who did worse things in the way of chemical experimentation! Unless we take the Girlfriends' advice, we have more than thirty-six weeks of worry ahead of us. The most common fear of retribution comes to those of us who were drunk or high when we conceived. What a double bind: You get loose enough to take the chance of getting pregnant, and then you spend your entire pregnancy wishing you had been stone-cold sober that night.

Eventually, God willing, the baby is born in robust good health. But for those of you who are not completely distracted by the outrageous experience of having a full-size baby come out of your insides, there will be a moment after that last push, or when the doctor reaches into your cesarean section, when you steel yourself for the possibility that you are going to be presented with a baby that looks more like Bubbles the Chimp than the Gerber baby. Believe your Girlfriends: The moment you hear your baby cry and you see its squishy little face, you will feel as if all the angels of heaven have smiled on you.

Then hold on to your seat, because you will be entering the Major Leagues of Worry. If you thought you obsessed about the little baby in your stomach, wait until you see how you wig out over the little baby you are now holding in your arms, who has immediately become the most important person in your household. (Remember how the Shirley MacLaine character in *Terms of Endearment* hovered over her baby's crib to see if she was breathing? When she wasn't sure she'd heard a breath, she gave the baby a good pinch that woke her up howling.)

You may think that this is hyperbole for the sake of drama, but you couldn't be more wrong. My Girlfriends and I were all convinced (primarily with our first babies) that we were keeping our newborns alive through the sheer force of our wills, that if we did not concentrate on them, they would stop breathing. We all held small mirrors under the baby's nose to see the moisture clouds that indicated respiration was indeed taking place. And those baby monitors that no mother can live without? Most of us kept the volume turned up so high in the early months that not only could we hear every breath and coo, we could hear the baby's fingernails grow.

Fear of Getting Ugly

Some women, such as my Girlfriend Shirley, have never been so beautiful and happy as when they are pregnant. They feel fulfilled as women, they glow with health, and they revel in their ripe, round figures. As I have said many times, "Goody-goody for them." Call me alienated from my role as a woman or as a reproducing creature, but I found the changes in appearance mildly disturbing at times, and sometimes downright horrifying. It's not that I look at pregnant women and find them unattractive. On the contrary—I think other pregnant women are adorable. I just have a hard time reconciling my own pregnant dimensions with the size 4 clothes in my closet.

I also wondered whether my husband would still find me sexy or, equally important, whether I would find myself sexy. The completely honest answer to both of these questions was no, but just as many Girlfriends and their mates find the whole experience deeply erotic. (More about this in the chapter "Sex and Pregnancy.")

I know it is boring and trite to condemn popular culture for promoting that thinness is next to godliness, but there is no denying that a pregnant woman may have an identity crisis in such a world. She may wonder whether she will lose her standing as a "babe" because she is growing a babe inside her. And as her clothes get too tight and her personal style gets challenged, she may wonder what she's even *supposed* to look like now. All pregnant women pray fervently that they will somehow be able to reclaim their former selves after the baby is born. But society sends mixed messages in this regard. On the one hand, you see a woman like Heidi Klum restored to her former beauty minutes after her baby is born, and you think that is what is expected of you. On the other hand is the universal comment "She looks so good . . . for having four children," as if having children were a justification for an appearance distinctly less than perfect. I must confess, however, that I will take a compliment any way I can get it, no matter how backhanded.

Fear of Turning into Your Mother

It is scary enough to make the transition from sweet young thing to MOTHER, but it is way scarier to contemplate turning into your *own* mother. It happens to all of us—we catch a glimpse of ourselves in the mirror, and whether it is the set of the jaw or the way we crinkle our eyes when we smile, we recognize someone in our face who is not us.

For many pregnant women, this transformation can lead to a full-fledged panic attack. Will you become a bossy, judgmental, rigid, and fretting person the way you always thought your mother was? You are sure that the mother you have always known never acted wildly and impetuously, never had sex in a Jacuzzi, and never dreamed of having an affair with Johnny Depp. (Or if she did, you never, ever want to hear a word about it.) That you may go from being Holly Golightly to PTA president is just too frightening to contemplate.

As you grow to love the baby that's inside you, you will have a new understanding of how much your mother must have loved you. You will begin to understand why she can't help herself when she butts into your life and is hypervigilant concerning your well-being. Just wait until the baby is two or three years old and you hear yourself yell, "Get down from there—you'll break your neck!" exactly as your mother used to. My own epiphany occurred when I caught myself spitting on a tissue and trying to clean my daughter's face before she walked into a birthday party.

Fear of Turning into Your Partner's Mother

I am not talking about the fear that you will transform into a physical replica of your mother-in-law. I am talking about changing from your partner's lover and friend into his asexual nurturer. Sometimes, in our determination to learn to mother before the baby is dumped in our laps, we start behaving like the mothers we grew up with, or worse, like the mothers our fellas grew up with. You'll know you are succumbing to this when you suggest that your guy wear a jacket because he might catch a chill, or when you begin making his dental appointments and offering to drive him.

This change is not usually made unilaterally, but rather with the cooperation of your partner. After all, who wouldn't want someone fussing over him? While most men maintain that their mother drives them crazy, they also love how their mother devotedly cared for them. You know how it goes: They want the Thanksgiving stuffing that their mother used to make, they want their shirts hung with the buttons facing the left of the closet, à la Mom, and they want you to make them a bed on the couch when they are sick, just as you-know-who always did.

Husbands encourage this mothering not just because they want to be babied, but because they, too, are intimidated by impending parenthood, and the only model they have for how mothers are supposed to act is their own mommy. It is amazing how many men develop an opinion about whether their wife is tidy enough or organized enough only when they learn that a baby is on the way.

Only one thing is more troublesome than being held to the romanti-cized standard of motherhood that your mate has been burnishing for the last twenty years, and that is being compared with his *first wife*. This is where you really must put your foot down. I don't care (and you shouldn't either) whether his first wife had her Christmas cards addressed by Hal-loween and made her own apple pie; she is no role model for you. If she were, her name would still be on the credit cards. Right?

Fear of Not Doing Pregnancy Right

Out of our overwhelming desire to be judged perfect, and the biological imperative to do everything we can to protect our unborn child from all the mishaps described above, we have set standards of proper behavior for pregnant women. If these standards were established individually between you and your doctor, I would applaud them. Unfortunately, many of us, through our inexperience and insecurity, buy into a whole litany of rules that are not only burdensome and unnecessary, but also guaranteed to make any woman feel inadequate.

If your own self-control and guilt aren't enough to keep you on the path of "perfect" parenting, you will soon learn that the world is filled with people who feel it is their responsibility to monitor your performance. The Girlfriends have dubbed these "oh so helpful" folks the Pregnancy Police. The only thing I hate more than a Pregnancy Police person is a MALE Pregnancy Police person. (As if a person without a uterus, or at least a medical degree, has any right to comment on how a pregnant woman lives her life.)

Pregnancy Police come from the same school as those complete strangers who feel free to pat your belly at the grocery store. Pregnancy Po-lice can be relied on to share all sorts of bullshit information. They always seem to know of a woman who had a fifty-hour labor and then needed an emergency C-section because the umbilical cord was wrapped around the baby's neck, or some such horror story. Of course the Pregnancy Police have an explanation for this crisis, and it almost always involves some shortcoming on the mother's part: either she was sleeping on her back rather than on her left side, or she took the epidural too early for the PP's taste, or some other bogus thing.

Pregnancy Police get tremendous satisfaction out of telling unsuspect-ing pregnant women that they should throw their microwave ovens into a toxic dump site, that they are being poisoned by the hidden formaldehyde in their mattresses, that they are exposing their baby to cancer by eating peanut butter, and that drinking a diet soda is tantamount to shooting heroin. The more distressed the mother-to-be becomes, the more fulfilled the Pregnancy Police feel. You would swear that they must have had perfect labors and deliveries and flawless children to have earned the credentials to tell you what you are doing wrong, but it never works out that way. It's like the child psychologist who lived next door to us when I was a kid: He was dispensing child-rearing advice on the phone in his study while his twins were setting the living room draperies on fire.

One of my Girlfriends remembers a time that she was in a beauty salon getting her roots touched up and a complete stranger approached her with a look of tremendous concern and inquired, "Don't you know you are not supposed to use chemicals on your hair when you are pregnant?" My Girlfriend, who already had half her head wrapped in aluminum foil with hair dye in it, went into an internal panic. She finished the coloring, but she left the salon near tears with the fear that she had ignorantly harmed her beloved baby. This hair-coloring business is something you should bring up with your doctor and decide for yourself, but my babies were all subjected to my hair dyeing in utero and they seem just fine to me.

My theory was this: If I had let my hair return to its natural brown and gray condition every time I was pregnant, my children might have been spared some indirect contact with chemicals, but they would also have been born to a single parent, because my husband would surely have left me after the first two inches of the "real me" had grown out. So if my kids didn't run the risk of biological imperfection, they would have run the risk of societal imperfection, along with their insane mother.

If my beauty-salon story sounds extreme, just wait until you run into the Pregnancy Police at a party or restaurant. God forbid if you should have a glass of wine with dinner or participate in a champagne toast, even with a notarized letter of permission from your doctor. The PP will either look witheringly at you or actually come up to you and lecture you about fetal alcohol syndrome. Almost all of the Girlfriends—none of whom, I hasten to add, drank more than a total of four or five glasses of wine or champagne over their entire pregnancy—found themselves more than once lamely trying to defend their imbibing to total strangers.

Naturally doctors will have their opinions about drinking during pregnancy, and I am neither condoning nor condemning drinking. I am just saying that pregnancy is hard enough. What with the societal stigmas against hot tubs, aspirin, coffee, and artificial sweeteners, not to mention your own compromised sex life and your comical physical proportions, a single drink late in pregnancy seems allowable, if not outright deserved. But, hey, I'm no doctor. Life is a series of calculated risks, and you and your doctor should work together to chart behavior that is healthy for the baby *and* livable for the mother.

One last hangout of Pregnancy Police is airports. They congregate near the security-clearance areas and will comment that you are nuking your baby if you walk through the X-ray machine. Now here, I have absolutely no complaints about their concern, but that is for personal reasons rather than any evidence I have regarding the danger of this kind of exposure to an unborn baby. I always made a big fuss about the danger of these X-ray machines so that I could be excused from passing through them. I was then hand-patted by a female security officer; and while I wasn't crazy about the patting part, I did like that I usually got to cut to the front of the line. For someone who is chronically late for flights, this could make or break my travel plans.

While we are on the subject of air travel, always check with the individual airlines to learn their policies regarding when they deem you "too pregnant" to be allowed on their planes. You know how fussy those flight attendants can be about labor and delivery on board. (And then, if you were Victoria Beckham, you'd have to name your child after the airline or its hub city.)

Fear of Being a Bad Mother

This fear usually comes from one of two possibilities: Either your own mother was so extraordinary, loving, patient, and selfless that you know you could never in a million years be as good a mother as she was, or your mother was such a selfish, neglectful, and undemonstrative person that you are terrified you may be genetically predisposed to act just like her. As in most aspects of pregnancy, there appears to be little middle ground.

Much as we would like to, we Girlfriends cannot predict what kind of mother you will be (although we have all the faith in the world in your mothering instincts). What we have all noticed is that pregnancy is the time to settle your issues with your own mother. Now is the time to look at your mother with a grown-up eye, as a woman with the same demands, insecurities, and hopes that you are feeling right now. You may emulate your mother, but *you are not your mother.* You have the opportunity to appraise your own childhood and pick and choose the parts that you want to share with your child and the parts you want to spare it.

Motherhood is a work in progress. You have nine (ten) months to prepare for some aspects of it, but you won't really understand what it feels like to be a mother until you have taken your child out of the hospital and into your home. It will be a love affair, but whether it will be love at first sight or a gradual thing varies from mother to mother. And you won't really know how good a mother you have been until your child sends thrilling and literate letters home from his Peace Corps job or sends postcards from his mobile home in the desert, where he collects roadkill and puts it in his freezer. You just love away and hope for the best—all the while coming to the stunning realization that this unbelievable love you have for your baby could just possibly be how your mom felt about you!

Fear of Labor and Delivery

See, I have saved the big one for last. This is the mother of all fears for a woman pregnant with her first child. At first, the fear of labor and delivery is really just the simple fear of pain. You have no doubt that it will hurt; a rudimentary understanding of simple physics will tip you off that a vagina that has never experienced anything larger than a super Tampax or a well-endowed fellow is going to balk at passing a watermelon through its dainty corridors. But you have no idea how *much* it will hurt. More than a bikini wax? More than a broken leg? More than a root canal?

After you have had enough time to hear the birth story of every woman you have ever met (roughly two weeks from the day you announce your pregnancy), your terror will expand to include the fear that you will be a wimp; the fear that you won't be able to push hard enough to get the baby out; the fear that you will make poopoo instead of pushing the baby out; the fear that you will faint or cry when they give you an IV (intravenous) needle; the fear that you will faint or cry, period; the fear that the epidural will hurt more than labor; or the fear that the anesthesiologist will have a bad aim and you will be paralyzed for life. We won't go into the details of labor and delivery and what they feel like here (there is an entire chapter devoted to them later), but we will discuss the essence of the Fear of Labor and Delivery, as we, your Girlfriends, see it.

The terror, in its most fundamental form, is that you will be in a vulnerable position, in pain, with your legs spread, scared of the creature that is insisting on coming out of you, AND NO ONE WILL DO ANYTHING TO SAVE YOU! Can't you just imagine yourself waddling into the hospital with the nagging suspicion that you are facing the trial of your life with a pitiful arsenal of Lamaze breathing, a Yanni cassette, and your hapless mate? You don't really consider other options because the Pregnancy Police (especially those Nazis in your prepared-childbirth class) tell you that you are doing it wrong if you vary from this prescription. To them I say, BULLSHIT! A healthy mother and baby, achieved under *any* conditions necessary, is the ultimate goal of labor and delivery.

We Girlfriends want to let you in on a secret. THERE IS NO AWARD CEREMONY FOR MOTHERS AFTER DELIVERY. No announcements are made over the loudspeaker; no medals are presented to those mothers who managed to deliver their children without pain medication, without crying, and without making a mess on the delivery table. First of all, few victors would emerge. Second, the other mothers in the audience would throw their hemorrhoid pillows at the medalists.

Here it is, Girlfriends: Epidurals are *great*. Cesareans can save lives and curtail unnecessary suffering. THERE IS NO SUCH THING AS A SECOND-CLASS BIRTH. Willingness to suffer or to put the baby or yourself in jeopardy, especially when you are frightened and tired, is a sign of questionable judgment, not heroism.

You have a choice: You can lie on a bed of nails to deliver your baby or you can lie on a bed of downy feathers. No matter what you choose, neither your doctor, your nurse, nor your baby will think any better of you for suffering because of some possibly misunderstood notion of what is best for your child. And trust us, your baby's father will think that you are a goddess for at least forty-eight hours after delivery, with or without medication, for enduring what looked at times like a horror show to him, to give him a child.

Keep this in mind: Those of us who took a little nip from the epidural tap are usually the life of the champagne celebration in our rooms after the baby is born, while our American Gothic counterparts are sound asleep with every capillary in their cheeks broken.

One last bit of advice about fear and worry: Learn to roll with it, because it doesn't ever really end. Even when you have the relief of holding a perfectly healthy baby in your arms after nine (ten) months of agitation, you are just warming up for serious worrying. You will wonder, "Is he getting enough to eat?" Or, "Is he eating too much and getting fat?" Then it's on to whether your child is the last one to be toilet trained in your Mommy and Me group, or whether she will make any friends. Then, as she gets even older and has plenty of friends, you worry whether those friends are good influences on your child—whether they take drugs, whether they're in a gang. Add to all that the abject terror all parents feel when their children are given driver's licenses and turned loose on America's highways, and you get a pretty good idea of why your own parents looked so distracted most of the time you were growing up. But I digress. . . .

6

You and Your Doctor

As YOU MAY already have deduced, the person you have known for years as your "gynecologist" transforms into your "obstetrician" on the day you find out you are going to have a baby. An obstetrician (or OB, in pregnancy lingo) is the person responsible for caring for a pregnant woman during gestation, delivery, and postpartum recovery. I guess that means that when they give you estrogen pills for menopause, they magically transform back into gynecologists.

Doctor or Midwife?

Nowhere is it etched in stone that you need a medical doctor to assist you in childbirth. A certified nurse-midwife, or lay midwife, can be the primary assistant to a delivering mother, either at the mother's home or at a birthing center that is usually affiliated with a doctor and is near enough by ambulance to a hospital should an emergency arise. Quite a few of the more forward-thinking doctors are now sharing their practices with certified nurse-midwives, and their patients see the doctor and the midwife on alternate visits. Since the vast majority of midwives are female, you get the Girlfriend factor built right into the relationship, and you may find yourself more comfortable asking certain questions of a midwife—such as "Is it normal to have so much gas?"—that you would never ask your doctor (most of whom still are men, as of this writing). There is also a belief that midwives might be less inclined than an overbooked obstetrician to hurry a delivery along through the use of pitocin or an eventual cesarean section.

My Girlfriend Kathy opted for a home birth with a nurse-midwife, and the midwife did everything from make her herb teas to walk with her in the hills outside her house to help bring on regular contractions. The nurturing and reassurance were extraordinary. Unfortunately, Kathy found labor longer, more painful, and more frightening than she had anticipated, and she ended up falling into the tiny backseat of her sports car and being whisked to a hospital to deliver her son. Her biggest disappointment was that because she had waited so long, the doctors decided not to give her any pain relief because it was time to push anyway.

I gleaned three lessons from Kathy's story. First, you can never get to the hospital too early, even if you end up spending the next twenty-four hours just walking the halls of the maternity ward. Second, save the home births, midwives, and underwater deliveries for second, third, and fourth babies. There is no way you can make an informed decision about how you want to manage your delivery until you have some realistic idea of what to expect. We Girlfriends guarantee that you will be surprised, perhaps pleasantly, perhaps not so pleasantly, but YOU WILL BE SURPRISED, even *after* reading this book. And third, never elect to have a child where you have no access to medication or, God forbid, real doctors.

You will tell yourself from now till labor begins that you intend to try delivering without an epidural, but I can't think of a Girlfriend who didn't take it when it was offered. Well, I take that back. My Girlfriend Jillian never took pain medication, but perhaps if her husband had not been there promising her jewelry if she could make it through, she, too, would have found the epidural a relief. (I wonder how it would go if she were to stand beside him with diamond cuff links while he was getting a vasectomy.) Nor was there any medication for Corki, whose baby had a heart problem that might adversely have been affected by it, or Amy, who labored too fast for the doctor to have time to get the epidural into her without slowing down her progress. But both Corki and Amy maintain that they would forever have been grateful for such medical intervention.

A postscript to this home delivery section: Childbirth is as messy as a pig slaughter. Why in the world would you want to sacrifice your beautiful sheets, not to mention your mattress, to such a thing? If you just can't stand the thought of going to a hospital, perhaps you should consider delivering at a four-star hotel; it's still cheaper than a hospital, and the food and maid service are infinitely better. (Wouldn't you just love to be in the room next door to that?)

How to Select Your Obstetrician

Did you notice how quickly we decided for you that a medical doctor will deliver your baby? We apologize if you think we are taking too much for granted, but that's what Girlfriends do. If you wanted something more statistical or analytical, you could have read any one of a million other books on pregnancy. Our job is to give you the inside scoop, based on what we tell each other, and our unanimous vote is to go for the traditional hospital birth with a godlike medical doctor for your first go-round on this birthing carousel.

Remember, we are creatures of popular culture; we revere doctors as if they were the heroes and heroines we grew up watching on TV. It's the *doctors* who are so honorably portrayed on everything from *Grey's Anatomy* to *General Hospital.* Poor, innocent midwives never have their own series, even on HBO. In fact, they were tried as witches in colonial Salem!

So how do you find that perfect person? Well, you can do one of two things: You can stick with the person who has heretofore been your gynecologist, the person who fitted you for an IUD and treated your yeast infections. Or you can pick a new doctor on the presumption that your needs are different now and that perhaps your gynecologist isn't necessarily the right person to get you through this pregnancy.

It can really be a mistake to think that your gynecologist of ten years must automatically deliver your child. Choosing the person who will deliver your baby is subject to different criteria than is choosing the person who does your Pap tests. There are many reasons to rethink your choice of doctors.

First of all, YOU SHOULD ASK YOUR GIRLFRIENDS WHAT THEY THINK OF THEIR OWN DOCTORS OR LOCAL DOCTORS. A real OB grapevine exists, and in most communities a few doctors' names come up over and over. I found my doctor when I was seated next to a Girlfriend of a Girlfriend in a salon. She had four children and positively glowed when she talked about her doctor. When another Girlfriend spoke of the same person in the same affectionate and reverent way, I knew I had found my man. I am still a satisfied customer.

It is also important to engage in some serious soul-searching to discover what kind of patient you are likely to be. If you are assertive and full of questions, you will need a doctor who doesn't resent making big allowances of time for you or who does email. If you are frightened about the entire prospect, you must absolutely select a doctor who is protective and understanding. Those eager to attempt a "natural" and "organic" pregnancy would be well-advised to find a doctor who not only supports your choice, but who has a special understanding of nutrition, environmental hazards, and treating colds with little more than hot water and lemon.

It is particularly important that you and your doctor share the same expectations for your birth experience. If you have your own reasons for wanting a C-section under any circumstances, then you and your doctor had better be in agreement about that from your first handshake. It also wouldn't hurt to discuss with your OB candidate your feelings and his regarding pain medication—not just *whether* you will get it, but *when* and *how much.*

When my first ultrasound showed pretty clearly that I was going to have a baby boy, I asked my Girlfriends with sons how they felt their doctors did on the circumcision. You may be surprised to learn, as I was, that it's the obstetrician, not the pediatrician, who does the tip clipping if you want your son circumcised in the hospital. If you don't think this is an important skill, just ask your mate's opinion. Some doctors seem to leave too much foreskin, some clip too far back, and it is still quite variable as to whether a topical anesthetic is used. Of course, not everyone circumcises these days, and most Jewish parents make a party of it.

Should Your Husband Be Consulted?

I don't think I know of a Girlfriend who ever consulted her partner about her choice of a gynecologist, unless, like my Girlfriend Kelly, she happened to be married to an obstetrician. Many of us have known our gynecologist far longer than we have our mates, and we never asked *them* what they thought of our boyfriends.

But we Girlfriends believe that when you're picking who will see you through this pregnancy, you should include your mate in the decision making. He will, after all, presumably be far more involved in the pregnancy and delivery than he was in your Pap tests. And for many reasons, it is critical that your partner feel almost as safe and comfortable with your doctor as you do. First, his child's entry into the world is in this doctor's hands. Second, your mate will presumably be at your side throughout most, if not all, of your labor, and it would be awfully nice if he liked the person who had his arm inside you up to his elbow. And third, he should feel as free as you do to call the doctor throughout the pregnancy to ask any questions he might have, or to secretly report any examples of your insanity.

Any suspicious or alarming symptoms that I experienced during pregnancy, I tearfully reported to my husband, and he called the doctor for me. When I started spotting, I was so panic-stricken that I couldn't form the words to speak on the phone, and my sweet husband called and described my condition. Labors, too, often tend to be reported to the doctor by the partners. Either the women are too involved with the contractions to carry on conversations (a reliable sign that a woman is in productive labor is her inability to get out a fluent sentence when a contraction strikes), or they are worried that they might not really be in labor. At a moment like this, a good partner will step in and remind you that you are entitled to call your doctor at any time, whether the baby is hanging down to your knees or not.

We are not saying this to alarm you, but it will blow your partner's mind even more than it blows yours when a baby emerges from your interior, since he's the one with the bird's-eye view, and he might really need someone to lean on. Let's not forget that your mate loves you very much and doesn't want anything bad to happen to you. Or more to the point, he doesn't exactly want to have you die in childbirth and leave him with this baby that he hasn't even met yet. He will insist on a doctor who'll guarantee that you will come out of this ordeal alive and well. Ultimately, however, your needs are paramount, and the final decision should be yours.

Male or Female?

Should your doctor be a man or a woman? It goes without saying that nearly any obstetrician in your community who has been recommended to you (and who is in good standing with the American Medical Association and hasn't been investigated on *60 Minutes*) will be competent to care for you during pregnancy and delivery of your baby. Whether you would prefer a female or a male doctor is a purely emotional decision. That is not to say, however, that it isn't a crucial one. We Girlfriends uniformly believe that your emotional safety and well-being are as critical to a successful birth as your medical support.

This is a time to throw political correctness aside and honestly appraise what type of person elicits your respect and trust and, in turn, trusts and respects you. This should probably be a private evaluation of your preferences, so that you are not swayed by a mother who thinks all good doctors are men or a sister who says she has never met a man who treated her as if her brain and spinal cord were connected. Do you prefer a male doctor because he seems fatherly and physically able to protect you from harm? Or perhaps you prefer a female doctor because she is more likely to empathize with you. As one Girlfriend asked, "Would you hire a mechanic who had never driven a car before?"

Then there is the whole issue of sexuality. Many of my Girlfriends, including Mindy and Maryann, were happy with their choice of female obstetricians because they felt less inhibited during physical exams and delivery, and they were freer to express their emotional concerns. These Girlfriends also mentioned the not unimportant fact that their husbands were reassured by their having female doctors for such an intimate relationship. In addition, there can be real pressure on a woman to maintain her attractiveness around men, since many of us learned this lesson early in life, and some aspects of pregnancy can make a woman feel less than attractive when exposed to her male doctor. This can create additional headaches, which is the last thing a pregnant woman needs.

On the other hand, you may ascribe to *my* philosophy that you grab your harmless pleasures where you can because pregnancy can be a long dry spell. The doctor who delivered three of my children is a man, and I had a great time flirting with him and taking special care with my appearance for my monthly visits. Of course, this doctor looks like Clark Kent, so I was not the only pregnant woman in town making a fool of herself. Especially in your last couple of months of pregnancy, your male doctor may be the only man on earth who is still interested in how you feel. A good many life partners have fallen by the wayside by that time. Remember, nine (ten) months of pregnancy will lead to about twelve visits to the doctor's office, and labor will involve hours of intense bonding between you and your doctor, so you had better pick carefully.

What Type of Practice?

Delivering babies is certainly the cheeriest medical specialty, but the hours suck. Except for scheduled inductions or C-sections, babies' births are unpredictable and often tedious and always seem to involve middle-of-the-night calls to the doctor. Chiefly for this reason, two or more doctors usually band together to divide up the number of sleepless nights they will have to endure and to try to get a vacation or two in each year.

With a group practice, each time you go for your monthly checkup, you are examined by a different member of the group. This ensures that you and all the doctors have at least shaken hands before you deliver a baby together. Then, when you go into labor and call your doctor, whichever member of the group is on call at that time will meet you at the hospital. So, not only can you look forward to the surprise of "It's a boy!" or "It's a girl!" but you can have the added surprise of hearing that "It's Dr. Hammill!" who will be attending your delivery.

For my first pregnancy, I chose a doctor in a group practice. My favorite doctor had the most seniority in the group and never got out of a warm bed to deliver a baby. That task always went to a newer member of the group who was still earning his or her stripes. Since I had a scheduled C-section, I not only had my favorite doctor on hand, but another doctor in the group, since two doctors usually attend this type of surgery. The other doctor was a woman my favorite doctor was dating at the time. It was really a sweet experience, watching the two of them work together. They worked with great professional skill, but they kept making goo-goo eyes at each other across my gored abdomen. (By the way, ten years later I learned that when their romance sputtered, the entire medical practice was blown to smithereens.)

My next three children were delivered by a doctor in a solo practice. About two of my pregnancies ago, he brought in a nurse-midwife to help take some of the pressure of the routine examinations off himself, but he did the delivering. In the rare event that he was unavailable to deliver a baby, he had an arrangement with a doctor in another practice to step in for him. Knowing what to expect, at least in this one respect, was a real blessing.

All of my doctor's patients ask two questions when they find out they are pregnant: "When is it due?" and "Will you be in town to deliver it?" One Girlfriend was so terrified that the doctor's wife would insist that he take a family vacation when the Girlfriend was due that she offered her parents' plush (and within-driving-distance-of-the-hospital) beach home to the doctor and his family just so she could keep him near.

This is not the place to speculate about the personal toll a solo practice takes on a doctor, since we are talking about someone you are going to have deliver your baby, not marry. But the decision about whether to select a doctor in a group or solo practice is important. It all boils down to this: In a group practice, you will never be sure who will join you in the delivery room until the moment arrives. On the other hand, a solo practitioner may have intestinal flu when you go into labor (or worse, be skiing with his family in Colorado), and you could end up having a stranger's hand on your cervix. At least in a group practice, you have shaken that hand.

Since this book was first written, solo practitioners have all but disappeared. Insurance just gets stingier and stingier, and it's hardly worth the paperwork and malpractice coverage costs for a single doctor to go it alone. More and more of us are in managed-care programs, whether we like them or not, and the doctors who will get us through gestation may be chosen for us. Still, if you do not feel comfortable with any of your caregivers, stand up for yourself and for your baby. You can request a different doctor until you are satisfied that you've found the one who makes you feel safe and understood.

Do Not Be Afraid of Your Doctor!

Doctors in general can seem too important, too busy, or too intimidating for us to bother with all of our questions and concerns. We might want to ask something of great importance to us, but worry that we will be wasting his or her time or, worse, *look stupid*. This applies when we are being treated for anything from chronic heart conditions to bunions, but it is particularly problematic when we are dealing with pregnancy.

A pregnant woman's relationship with her doctor is uniquely complex because, in the vast majority of cases, she is not *sick*. Except for supervision of her condition and the growth and development of her pregnancy, the pregnant woman offers relatively little to treat medically. The only *cure* for her condition is delivery, and until that thrilling time, she and her doctor are basically waiting for the proverbial watched pot to boil. This basic condition of good health is usually cause for gratitude on the pregnant woman's part, but it can make her feel sheepish when she needs some emotional support or reassurance from her doctor. Since our view of doctors is that they are in the business of saving lives, we are often reluctant to intrude on that mission unless we are convinced that we are at death's door.

My Girlfriend Whitney sat for nearly twenty hours with another Girlfriend who was going through an early miscarriage. The Girlfriend suffering the miscarriage had been through this ordeal before, and since she knew what was happening to her physically, she saw no reason to bother her doctor with her news until it was over. What she needed was reassurance (a good painkiller wouldn't have been a bad idea, either), but she was reluctant to be unnecessarily demanding of her doctor's valuable time.

I am sure her doctor would agree with me when I say *this was a big mistake!* All good obstetricians are fully aware of the emotional nurturing that a pregnant woman requires, and if they aren't, you should drop them like hot potatoes. I once had a gynecologist who was treating me for infertility (can you believe it, four children later?). One day he walked into the examining room and asked, "How are you?" I started to cry and say that I was feeling pretty blue and frustrated. He did an about-face and called over his shoulder as he walked out the door, "I will send in a nurse to talk to you." Not only did I immediately stop seeing him, but I wrote him a pointed letter. Most gratifying of all was my pleasure in trashing this doctor all over the Girlfriends' Grapevine. Hell hath no fury . . .

If *The Girlfriends' Guide* accomplishes little else, I will be satisfied if it succeeds in encouraging you to get your money's worth out of your relationship with your doctor. Trust me when I tell you that it takes a long time to get over a disappointing pregnancy. If you feel ill-prepared, frightened, or slighted in any way, you will still be talking about it twenty years from now. I have a Girlfriend who still talks about how inadequate she felt during labor, and I think it was her doctor's job to bolster her confidence. Women who end up with C-sections when they had their heart set on a "natural" childbirth can be filled with grief, unless they are confident that it was a mutual decision and that it was the best thing to do. So go ahead and call your doctor or go visit him or her whenever the urge arises, because I promise you that you are no more neurotic or insecure than the rest of us. And if she can't take your call at that moment, leave a message; if you don't hear back by six o'clock that evening, call when you wake up in the morning and begin pestering her office. As Glenn Close said in *Fatal Attraction,* "I won't be ignored!"

What If You Think You Are Falling in Love with Your Doctor?

Sometimes, the combination of dependency and admiration that you feel for your doctor may make you think that you are falling in love. Relax—it is strikingly common for a pregnant woman to fall in love with her doctor, especially when her doctor is a man, but either way. Perhaps it is a form of hostage identification syndrome, as when Patty Hearst fell in love with her Symbionese Liberation Army kidnapper. The theory goes that utterly helpless people identify and develop a relationship with their captor because that person is all that stands between them and certain death. Sounds about right for a woman pregnant with her first child and her relationship with her doctor, don't you think?

You may also get a crush on your doctor because you are desperate for any kind of attention, and your obstetrician joins you in your obsession at least once a month. (As unique and special as your pregnancy is, it tends to lose its fascinating and compelling aspects to everyone but your mother and you about halfway through. And unfortunately, a pregnant woman's need for attention is as deep as the Grand Canyon.) I hate to be so blunt, but it is important for you to remember YOU DID NOT INVENT PREGNANCY, AND EVENTUALLY YOU WILL HAVE TO RESORT TO PAYING PEOPLE TO REMAIN CAPTIVATED BY YOUR CONDITION. Your friends have their own lives, which will occasionally distract them from your crucial project, and, if your mate is like mine, even he will eventually tire of waking up to touch your belly every time the baby moves. Your doctor, however, will continue to be solicitous and inquiring right up until the end—assuming, of course, that you have selected your obstetrician based on *The Girlfriends' Guide* criteria. Plus, he or she will eventually become the only person you encounter who does not irritatingly ask you, "Haven't you had that baby yet?"

7

Prenatal Tests

THERE ONCE WAS a time when the only medical test routinely given to a woman suspecting she was pregnant resulted in a dead rabbit. It's true—the old-fashioned way of diagnosing early pregnancy was to administer a serum of the woman's blood to a rabbit, and if the rabbit died, the woman was officially pronounced pregnant (and ineligible for PETA membership, unless she had a fur coat to swap for the rabbit . . . just kidding!). There wasn't much testing after that, just a lot of weighing and the occasional check for iron deficiency.

Welcome to the twenty-first century, Girlfriend, because nowadays you may have been testing for pregnancy-related issues even before you conceived. If you used an ovulation-predictor kit, you're already accustomed to conducting toilet science. If you've had a bit of fertility treatment thrown in, you've been ultrasounded and blood-tested regularly. We are a society that is obsessed with our biology, and few conditions are more lab-friendly than pregnancy. You can even test for that at home now, and most of us do, but that doesn't stop us from testing again at the doctor's office, just for a reality check. Depending on your age and some other factors, such as how comprehensive your medical insurance is, a variety of medical procedures might be recommended or even required of you during the next few months.

Another Disclaimer

Once again, let me make it clear that this is not a medical book. My purpose is simply to make you aware of the basics of pregnancy and describe them for you as your Girlfriend. Think of this chapter as an introductory foreign-language course, where you learn how to ask where the bathroom is and how to order dinner so that you don't look like a complete imbecile. Once you get the lingo, you'll know how and when to ask your doctor or practitioner for the real information.

The following list is not to be considered comprehensive in any way (since there's some new test or technology every year or so); it is just the collection of the Girlfriends' most commonly experienced tests and procedures. Having more or fewer than these tests is not in itself a cause for worry. If you have more, it doesn't mean you have more problems, and if you don't have them all, don't curse your health-care provider because you think you're getting gypped—these tests and screenings are just on the menu for you and your doctor to consider.

The Pregnancy Test

There are basically two kinds of early-pregnancy tests: the kind that uses blood and the kind that uses urine. Both of them detect the hormones that indicate that you've got a little critter in your belly who is already making himself known by excreting certain chemicals and making your body react. Oh, and by the way, neither of these tests uses injections into any of earth's creatures. The urine tests are so reliable, almost 100 percent when the result is positive, that your doctor's office will probably use a test much like the one you already took in your bathroom. Occasionally a blood test is done to confirm the pregnancy, especially if the doctor wants more information about all your hormone levels to see if you're mixing the right cocktail of hormones to maintain a pregnancy.

They Vant Your Blood

More commonly, the blood tests pregnant women get early on are to check a variety of things that will provide necessary information about your health and that of your baby. They all require a "venous puncture," meaning they put the band around your upper arm and stick a skinny needle into a promising vein. It stings, sure, but it's the freak factor and occasional light-headedness that upsets some of my Girlfriends. Just turn your head and breathe a deep cleansing breath and it will be all over. Plus, you'll get a Band-Aid to show off for the rest of the day. It's usually just one stick, and then they fill up several vials with your blood to send off to the lab, so stay calm. Here's what they will probably be testing for:

1. Your blood type (do you even know it?) and to see if you're Rh-positive or -negative. If you are negative and your baby is positive, your pregnancy will require special care to protect the baby from anemia. Ask your doctor for a full explanation if you really want to know.
2. To see if you are anemic.
3. To check for STDs.
4. To see if you've had rubella (German measles).
5. To see if you have hepatitis B, a liver virus.
6. To see if you have HIV.

Remember, *all* of these things, if detected, can be dealt with safely; you may just need to work more closely with your doctor to take care of yourself and your precious little baby.

Vaginal Cultures (Yuck!)

During the first prenatal visit, in addition to the blood test, a Pap test is usually done. You know the drill: stirrups, speculum, and a giant Q-tip to swab off some gunk and a few cells from your cervix, to check for STDs and anything yeasty up in there. These samples are put in some petri dishes or on slides and sent off to a lab. You probably won't hear anything about them unless there's a suspected problem.

While he or she is down there, your doctor will also take a gander at your cervix, which is the little tunnel between your vaginal canal and your uterus. (So few of us really know what exactly IS down there!) A good sign is when the cervix appears tightly closed and is beginning to take on the pinkish hue that indicates there's a good blood supply down there. After the first visit there will be few, if any, more vaginal exams during pregnancy. I think the feeling is to let sleeping dogs lie.

Here's Your Cup, There's the Bathroom, What's Your Hurry?

Get used to this one, Girlfriend, because it's going to be the greeting you will receive every time you visit your doctor or practitioner. Gradually, you will lose any inhibitions you may have about wandering around with a cup of your own body waste. (Keep in mind what we told you earlier about losing your aim as your labia swell. You might want to *watch* the stream for a second or two before pausing to put the cup in it.) A nurse or lab tech will set it next to all the other cups, and while you're wondering why one is yellower than yours and another is light as straw, she will put a test strip in it and you'll probably walk away, never to think about it again until next month.

This test checks the levels of protein and sugar in your urine. While some sugar in the urine is completely normal, too much can be a sign of diabetes. (Later, a more specific test can determine if you are at risk for gestational diabetes.) Protein in the urine might indicate a urinary tract infection (which will probably come as no surprise since the discomfort should have tipped you off), kidney problems, or, late in pregnancy, if you have high blood pressure, which can result in preeclampsia, aka toxemia. (Again, talk to a doctor about this. All I remember when my Girlfriend Jamie had this was that her hands, feet, and face got swollen as if she'd eaten too much salt and was retaining water. She delivered by C-section after a brief hospital stay, and the baby was perfection, and the mom was, too, after she calmed down.) Keep in mind, my sweet, all of this stuff can safely be handled, and you and your baby will most likely be just dandy.

Blood Pressure

Another feature of every prenatal visit will probably be the taking of your blood pressure. This is a fairly pleasant little ritual that isn't invasive in any way. My best advice is to stop chattering away to the nurse while she's doing the test or else you'll distract her in her counting, and she'll have to start all over again. This might not be an imposition on you, but it could annoy her. The reason for this test is that pregnant women have a greater risk of high blood pressure (and who wouldn't, under these circumstances?), and we all know that high blood pressure can lead to preeclampsia/toxemia.

Ultrasounds/Sonograms: You Say Tomato and I Say Tomahto

Unless I'm missing a fine distinction here, these are the same thing. Maybe the grams are the photos and the sounds are the images on-screen, but we're splitting hairs. If you ask my Girlfriends and me, this jolly test is like a porthole to paradise. Seeing something early in my pregnancy they told me was a baby, but looked like a lima bean with a little heartbeat, convinced me that I really was going to be a mommy. Up until that point, I'd often suspected that it was a dream or some terrible mistake. I cried like a baby (as the old pun goes).

The way ultrasounds work is that a dildo-like thing is placed in your vagina (they even put a condom on it and some lubricating gel, but don't get too excited, Girlfriend) or its rectangular cousin is placed on your belly (yes, you get gel then, too, and it's warm in the nicest doctors' offices) to make sound waves that can be translated into images we get to see. The doctor or technician performing this likes to get a look from several angles, so he or she will be moving the transducer, as the gel-coated thing is called, around a lot. No problem over your belly, but a tad uncomfortable when it's inside you. Not to worry, however, because you'll be transfixed by the staticky image on-screen. Besides, this is a good time to try out those Lamaze breathing techniques everyone raves about.

For a good ultrasound image early in pregnancy, you will have to drink a lot—and I mean *a lot*—of water for the transducer to pick up good sound, especially if they are using the tummy transducer. The vaginal one requires much less water, and it's worth asking in advance which they will be using or if they will use both. The doctor or technician will tell you if you should come for the ultrasound with a full bladder. Do you have any idea how much water it takes to fill your bladder, Girlfriend? Judging from my experience, it took more water than I've ever drunk in my life. It was the first time in my life that I got nauseous and wanted to barf from drinking water. My teeth were floating by the time I had my first ultrasound, and I was terrified I was going to lose control and drown everyone in the room. Later in pregnancy, when your baby is floating around like a sea horse in an aquarium, the ultrasound will not require you to drink still more.

The technology of ultrasounds is so fine now that the most experienced doctors can not only count the chambers of the heart and inspect the spine, but they can measure the fetus's neck and its thighbone for any evidence of a genetic irregularity. And if the baby is feeling saucy, it might just reveal its private parts to you. If you see a penis, don't jump to conclusions, however, because even baby girls look to the untrained eye like they have a penis. If you don't want to know your baby's gender, tell your doctor and ultrasound tech right away so they don't spill the beans and can tell you when to look away from the screen. *Keep* reminding them, too, because my Girlfriend Garbo's doctor started referring to her baby as "him" by about her seventh month, and sure enough, she had a boy. It's the little slips that we moms catch and obsess over.

This test is also the most certain way of knowing, before they actually arrive, if twins or more are in there. A couple of years ago, *Oprah* had a woman on who had IVF and had two fertilized eggs put back into her body. BOTH of them divided into two babies and she gave birth to two sets of identical twins! Get out! Anyway, this is something that can be detected through ultrasound because the placentas and sacs can be inspected pretty thoroughly. Even those of us who say we "want to be surprised" will need a month or three to adjust to the prospect of having an entire family in one gestation. Plus, as a rule, doctors HATE surprises, so they'll want to know right away.

One of the most precious sights a mommy-to-be can see is the image of her baby moving around or, still more enchanting, sucking its thumb just like a *real* baby. These are the photos and, occasionally, videos that you'll be showing your friends and family for weeks. In fact, you'll probably still have the little Polaroid picture stuck up on your refrigerator door with a magnet months after your baby is born.

Some health plans don't regularly cover the cost of ultrasounds, but you'll probably get at least one around the sixth or seventh month, and if your age or your doctor's suspicion that some other situation requires a closer look warrants it, you'll get at least one more. I would have liked to look every month, or even every week—so I can kind of understand why Tom Cruise bought his own ultrasound machine for his baby with Katie Holmes. Still, for a Scientologist who espouses "silent birth," that's a lot of sound waves banging around in there. Hey, his machine isn't busy right now; maybe you can go over and use it sometime.

Glucose Tolerance Test: "Sugar Sugar, Honey Honey, You Are My Candy Girl"

Even if you don't have diabetes in real life (as opposed to these nine [ten] months of tripping), you may develop gestational diabetes. The good news about this kind is that it almost always goes away after delivery. It's important to have this test because gestational diabetes is fairly common, especially with the higher incidence these days of type 2 diabetes in our country. If your doctor says you have it or are on your way to getting it, you will have to watch your diet and strictly follow your OB's directions, but you and your baby will probably be fine. If you don't do as you're told, or even if you do, you might end up with a large or heavy baby, which could have you delivering by C-section (or wishing you were).

The first thing you must know about this test is that refrigerating the sugar substance they're going to make you drink makes it taste a lot less awful. Your doctor may tell you that, or you may be given the sample from their refrigerator, but if no one says anything, ask them if you can take your drink home and keep it in your fridge for a day before drinking it for the test. The cold seems to numb your taste buds, and my Girlfriends and I swear by it, even if it's only in our heads.

The drink comes in a little bottle about the size of an old-fashioned Coke. It tastes like a soft drink that has lost its carbonation and has had an extra half-cup of sugar mixed in. Whatever it tastes like to you, it won't be good. You may be tempted to chug it all down and get it over with as fast as you can, but the Girlfriends and I lovingly suggest you take it easy and break it up into several sips (OK, gulps). This test requires you to drink the stuff on an empty stomach for an accurate reading, so if this is the first food to hit your stomach in twelve hours, your tummy may revolt and toss it all back up. If you don't like vomiting and you don't want to drink the foul stuff twice, taking a couple of minutes to down it might be a good idea.

After an hour, they will take blood from your arm to see how you are processing the massive sugar intake. You probably won't know right away, so your job will be done then, unless they want a second blood test in another hour. At this point you will want some real food in your belly, so come prepared with a sandwich, trail mix, or fruit. You probably won't be craving anything sweet, so aim for protein and some good carbs (hey, they're all good to me, but I'm not a nutritionist either). Just don't go for the salt fix of chips or fries because no water-retaining Girlfriend needs *more* sodium in her diet.

Alpha-Fetoprotein Test

This test finds out if you have a higher than average risk of having a baby with certain birth defects such as Down syndrome or spina bifida. Don't freak; most states require you to have this test, so you aren't being singled out for anything. The test consists of yet another vein puncture, but they don't take much—besides, you must be getting used to this by now. It's usually done when you are about fifteen to eighteen weeks pregnant. The blood is sent to a lab, and the results are shared with your doctor and often your state health department (at least that's how I understand it). You won't hear anything for about a week, so your work is done when they give you a Snoopy Band-Aid.

Occasionally, there are low or high levels of the baby's protein in your blood; low could mean one thing, and high could mean another. (See, your baby is already taking over your body and pouring its waste out through you.)

When this happens, you may get a call from the doc to go back in for another test. If this happens to you, DON'T PANIC. These results are usually considered *indicators* that there *might* be a problem—they are not usually the final word. My Girlfriend Mindy got a low level of fetal protein in her blood test, and since this sometimes coincides with Down syndrome, she was called back to her doctor's office. We were all weak with fear and near panic, but an amnio negated that result, and her baby girl was born healthy and at her due date. Keep this in mind, because all of us are prone to irrational fears about our babies, even before we meet them face-to-face, and yet they almost always turn out fine.

Amniocentesis

Amnios, as we vets refer to them, test the genetic health of your unborn baby (and its gender, too, if you're curious). They are not routinely performed, but for mothers who will be thirty-five or older when they deliver, they are usually prescribed and paid for by your insurance or HMO. This is because we older gals have a higher incidence of babies with chromosomal defects such as Down syndrome, because our eggs are getting a bit tired. (That's Girlfriendspeak for "Ask your genetic counselor.") It is also prescribed for younger mommies with genetic problems in their family or in that of the father.

If you are a candidate for amnio, you will probably be scheduled at around sixteen to eighteen weeks gestation. It is performed by doctors, in their office if they have the machinery, or referred out to a lab and a doctor who specializes in this procedure. They will use an ultrasound to carefully determine exactly where the baby is and NOT put the needle there. They are aiming for the amniotic fluid, which they draw out for the screening. If you open your eyes to look, you will see that the fluid is straw-colored and pretty clear. Floating in that water are cells the fetus has sloughed off and doesn't need anymore. Those cells are sent to a lab, where they will be cultured to grow for a couple of weeks or so and analyzed by the pros.

Are you still reading, Girlfriend? Many of us have had to sit down and put our head between our legs at this point of the description. When you have recovered and can continue reading, we rush to reassure you THE AMNIO WILL NOT BE AS BAD AS YOU'RE IMAGINING AT THIS MOMENT.

Almost everyone who is advised to get an amnio is beyond frightened or numb with denial. I know this fear up close and personal: In my first pregnancy, which took over three years to achieve, I was lying on the exam table with my belly draped and swabbed with that brown disinfectant they use, and I chickened out. Yup, I got up from the table crying, wiped the brown stuff off, and got dressed while whimpering something incoherent to the doctor and to me. I drove home still whimpering, and I never returned to have the test.

We were lucky that time, but I never skipped the test again with the other three babies, and I cannot stress this enough to you: Never let fear prevent you from getting the information you need for your health and the baby's. Pony up, cowgirls, we can face this together.

The reasons we are terrified of amnios are threefold. First, with the long needle they use, we think it will hurt like a son of a gun. Second, our genetics counselors or OBs have legally been obligated to tell us that there is a small chance of the test itself harming the fetus or causing the miscarriage of a healthy fetus. And third, and most agonizing of all, if the amnio tells us, God forbid, that our baby is genetically abnormal, we would have to decide whether to terminate the pregnancy.

This is one of the most horrific decisions a couple will ever have to make, and the prospect of facing it is brain-twisting. After all, if you are absolutely against abortion, why get an amnio in the first place, unless you feel forewarned is forearmed? Or if, like most of us, you are unsure where you stand on terminating a pregnancy, hearing that your fetus is not viable will quickly force you to decide.

There, now that I have you ready to slit your wrists, let me rush to reassure you that your odds are incredibly good of having a perfectly normal baby, although *you* may never be the same . . . I know I'm not. Age forty and above can be more risky, and that's just to say you should undertake it with information and a good doctor. Even then, however, the odds are still overwhelmingly in your favor. As my father told me when I fretted to him about my fourth pregnancy at the age of thirty-nine, "I would play your odds at the racetrack any day of the week."

In all likelihood, all amnio will do for you (besides tell you whether to pick blue or pink onesies) is relieve you of some of your phantom worries about your unborn baby. I wish I could tell you that it makes the rest of your pregnancy worry-free, but it doesn't work that way. After you have eliminated Down syndrome and other *testable* genetic abnormalities from your worry list, you will simply and certainly replace them with fears of cleft palates (although these can often be detected in a thorough ultrasound), strawberry birthmarks, and a genetic marker for male-pattern baldness. Remember this: Pregnancy is the beginning of the slippery slope of worry, down which you will careen for the rest of your life.

So, now let's talk about whether it hurts. The answer is, yes, a little bit. (I would like to interject here that, having given birth several times, I chuckle when I speak of pain, so this is for you *virgins*. After you have delivered a baby, pain may take on another meaning . . . and a lot of pride.) More than being painful, the amnio rates high on the Creeps Factor Index. Some doctors offer a shot of novocaine in your belly before the amnio needle. Others will say, "Why take two needles when you can do it with just one?"

Here's why, Girlfriends: because the novocaine needle is about two inches long and has the circumference of a hair. The anmio needle is about seven inches long and is substantially thicker than the other. I can't speak for everyone, but I liked the sense of security that the novocaine instilled in me. I was in the room holding my Girlfriend Amy's hand during her amnio, and she went straight for the big needle and didn't flinch. Now, Amy is pretty brave, but other Girlfriends have told me that they opted to skip the novocaine and go straight for the big shot, too. Really, the only place with any nerves to detect pain is your skin; once they get in there, you can't really feel much, except fear and light-headedness. But that's just me: If someone is offering an easier, softer way, count me in, even if it's all in my tiny little head.

After the amnio, you will probably feel much as you did when you entered the room, except a lot more relieved and extremely tired from the emotional ordeal. You doctor will tell you to go home and get in bed, and we Girlfriends emphatically agree. In fact, we suggest that you do that *whenever* you feel tired or weepy or overwhelmed—just bring your phone in with you so you can call your Girlfriends for support. I don't know what a day in bed does for the baby, but I suspect the doctors want your needle prick to heal before you resume your power walking. I do know from experience, however, that a day of soaps and *Dr. Phil* has amazing recuperative powers. Take advantage of this doctor's order to take to your bed, Girlfriend, because this is one of the few days you can cocoon without a twinge of guilt.

Chorionic Villus Sampling (CVS—and We Don't Mean the Pharmacy)

This is what I elected to do for genetic screening instead of amnios with my younger kids. As I've confessed, I walked out on my amnio with my first pregnancy. After the genetics counselor told me that, at my age (then thirty-four), I had a 1 in 200 chance of a genetic abnormality, and there was, at that time at least, a 1 in 200 chance of the amnio causing me to miscarry, I wussed and walked.

Amnios are still the more common genetic screening procedure, but I have my own little conspiracy theory about that: I think that so many OBs invested time and money in the skills and technology to perform amnios in their office (and let's face it, there's a big profit incentive there, Girlfriends) that they don't refer out to the doctors who specialize in CVS. This is simply my thinking on the matter, but my Girlfriends tell me I'm a cynic, so feel free to ignore everything I just said. Besides, it's only natural to want to have such a sensitive test performed by a doctor you know and love and trust, rather than a total stranger. And with doctors becoming an underpaid class as insurance evaporates and malpractice suits rise to the point of lunacy, I honor any opportunity for a doctor to make a profit *somewhere*. OK, I'm stepping down from my soapbox.

CVS tests for most of the same genetic abnormalities as amnio, with the exception of neural-tube defects such as spina bifida, and determines the gender of the baby, too. It involves the same genetic counseling. I preferred it because CVS is performed at eleven or twelve weeks of pregnancy and the results can come back as quickly as twenty-four hours later. One of the biggest drawbacks of the amnio is that you are about five months pregnant before you get the results. By that time, you are halfway through your pregnancy and already feeling the baby kick, so the prospect of having to terminate the pregnancy could be particularly excruciating. With a

CVS, however, you can have the test and the results several weeks before anyone really even needs to know you're pregnant. That can be a blessing, Girlfriend—because the last thing a couple needs at this difficult time is an audience, especially one that feels it has a vote. Whatever you decide, you can make the decision without the approval or disapproval of people who have never been faced with such a crisis.

A CVS is done in conjunction with an ultrasound. Since it is done early in pregnancy, you will need to drink a lot of water before the procedure (see "Ultrasounds/Sonograms" above). The tech assisting my doctor actually did an advance ultrasound on me to see if I was too full and my bladder was blocking the view of my uterus. Since mine was, twice, I was sent to the bathroom to release some. Only through heroic self-control did I not just empty my entire bladder at that moment, but she gave me a cup to measure how much I let go and told me not to pee a drop more than that. Can you believe the faith she had in me?

After the assisting tech rechecked the gestational age of the fetus and that it had a heartbeat (my favorite part), the doctor joined us. Yes, my legs were in stirrups, *again,* and as with a Pap test, the doctor used a speculum to open my garage door and keep it open. He dunked those giant Q-tips into Betadine to disinfect my vaginal canal and cervix. That was actually the most uncomfortable part for me; it felt as if I were having my insides scrubbed with a Turkish towel. When I was scrupulously clean, the assisting tech used an external (hence all the water you have to drink) ultrasound transducer to locate the baby and its chorionic villi, which are the tissues that will develop into the placenta. Using the ultrasound picture as his guide, the doctor inserted a tiny, thin plastic tube through the cervix and into the uterus. Then he sucked out a tiny portion of the villi. It didn't hurt, and because no needles were in sight, I didn't get too creeped out. Besides, as with amnio, the ultrasound pictures on the monitor are so enthralling that you tend to forget everything else that's going on. CVS can also be performed through a needle in the belly like amnio, just earlier. If you have bleeding or spotting in early pregnancy, your doctor may feel more comfortable waiting for an amnio, because there is a higher risk of bleeding with a CVS.

After it was over, I went home and crawled into bed with *The Price Is Right* and Susan Lucci and loved every moment of it. I think I slept most of the time. And yes, with my last CVS, I did experience bleeding and I *freaked.* I thought that my desire to have the earlier test had endangered my pregnancy and I was being punished for lacking faith and patience. But when your doctor is experienced with this procedure (and you should ask how many of these he or she has performed), the risk seems to be the same as with amnio.

All in all, 95 percent of all women having amnio or CVS will go on to have a healthy baby, so don't work yourself into a lather over this—although almost all of us do.

nonstress Test

The name of this test has nothing to do with *your* emotional state when it is taken. It refers, rather, to the baby being electronically monitored in its natural, nonstressed condition of growing and living the life in your big belly. Your belly will indeed be huge if and when you have this test, because it is generally used to check on babies who are near term or past their due date, just to make sure that they are still groovin' in the womb.

This test is usually performed by someone other than the doctor, since the doctor rarely wants to sit around watching your baby's heartbeat repeatedly graphed on endless strips of paper for up to an hour, riveting though you may think it is. The nurse or technician will put a fetal-monitor belt around your tummy with the microphone thingy as close to the baby's heartbeat as she can get it. Most likely, she will then turn around and walk out of the room, leaving you to stare at the graphing paper or fall asleep or bite your cuticles. (This is good preparation for what often happens to Girlfriends in labor.) The point of this test is to see if the baby's heartbeat responds properly to its own movement and to any contractions your exercising uterus may be doing. As you approach or pass your due date, your doctor may want to make sure that the baby isn't overstaying its welcome and doesn't need to be encouraged to leave.

The odds are good that you will never have this test, but I mention it because I don't want you to worry if your doctor suggests it. Also, many of my Girlfriends and I got overly attentive to our almost-born baby's movements and rushed to the doctor's office when we could swear the baby was dead because we hadn't felt it move in twenty-four hours. We were all put on the monitor and left the office reassured that our babies were moving as much as they could, under the tight circumstances. My babies, by the way, always fell asleep during the nonstress test, and I was invariably given fruit juice to give the little critters a sugar rush and make them move. One time, the nurse put an electric zapper to my belly to shock my baby into activity. It wasn't harmful to the baby or me, but it buzzed mightily, like those practical-joke things you shake somebody's hand with. Eventually I was accepting of my lazy babies because a lazy baby can be a mellow baby, and when you have four kids, you begin to admire mellowness as a character trait.

Weighing In

OK, so stepping onto a doctor's scale doesn't qualify as a prenatal test. So sue me. Still, you will be weighed every single time you visit your obstetrician, and this is part of monitoring both your health and that of your baby. So I say it stays *right* here in this chapter of the book, and you can't make me move it.

If there is no *real* crisis with your pregnancy, weighing in every month can be the most painful medical procedure that you will be asked to endure. I dreaded this part of an otherwise lovely visit to my doctor because I consistently gained more weight than certain *other* pregnancy books told me was correct. I got so sick of it, I eventually wrote my own book to calm us all down, and here it is. When I only gained one or two measly pounds between visits, I would be so proud and happy that I practically danced out of the office, but when I gained six pounds between visits, I felt that I'd got an F for the day and was a loser because I couldn't control myself and my urges and I was a big fat pig.

Eventually, after the first two or three pregnancies, I noticed something that my Girlfriends also pointed out to me: We all tended to put on the same amount of weight with each pregnancy, give or take a pound or two, regardless of our eating habits and level of physical activity. Sure, with our first gestational journeys many of us are so excited with the free pass to life's buffet that we overindulge, but the weight gain of second and third pregnancies seems to be encoded in our DNA. In other words, whether your body's style is to get huge eating a cube of cheese three times a day or to gain only ten pounds on a diet of protein shakes and pasta, it will probably stay true to that style with each pregnancy.

Basically, if you steer clear of Boston cream pies and eat less than a loaf of bread a day, and you make an effort to fulfill your baby's and your nutritional needs, you're doing a fabulous job. I say this over and over, but it's worth restating: There are no prizes for perfect pregnancies and deliveries, so stop competing. Besides, if there's a problem, you can be sure that your doctor will tell you. Just between us, Girlfriend, I gained thirty-five pounds with every baby and I lied about my pre-pregnancy weight so it didn't look so dramatic. "Nine months up, nine months down," I always say.

8

Exercise and Pregnancy

I HAVE ALWAYS thought of pregnancy as divine permission not to exercise. For that reason, this chapter is even more opinionated than the others. It will focus on some exercises that you have never even dreamed about, and it will fly in the face of all the current notions that a woman should be able to grow a baby and run a marathon simultaneously. It's *my* book and it's *my* opinion, so there! Don't get me wrong: I am not anti-exercise. In fact, I am quite keen on doing all sorts of fitness activities. When I am not pregnant, I jog, I lift weights, and I engage in whatever other fad is popular in my neighborhood, from kickboxing to pole dancing. But I am a firm believer in the maxim IF YOU WANT TO DO SOMETHING WELL, GIVE IT AS MUCH ATTENTION AS YOU POSSIBLY CAN. In other words, you are trying to grow a healthy baby without also sustaining too much damage to yourself, and that deserves all the attention you can give it. Working, taking care of your other kids, and doing all the other things that constitute living your life will be distractions enough (especially when you are lugging around an extra thirty or forty pounds). If you find yourself with extra time on your hands, like my Girlfriend Shannon, who is an actress and who was unable to work once her pregnancy started showing, spend it needlepointing a Christmas stocking, organizing your photo albums, or creating new playlists for labor and delivery on your iPod. I guarantee you that you will never have time to do those things again once the baby is born.

I can just feel the controversy that will arise over these statements. Doctors, fitness gurus, and women who successfully exercised throughout their pregnancies are going to come looking for me, their water bottles poised for combat. I feel so strongly about this that I am willing to take them on. I realize that a large number of you will want to dismiss me out-

Here are the biggest reasons why we Girlfriends don't think you need to keep up your gym membership while you are pregnant:

1. You Will Be Too Tired.
2. You Won't Look like Yourself in the Harsh Gym Mirrors.
3. You Will Get Fat Anyway.
4. Exercise Will Not Help You in Labor or Delivery in Any Way.
5. You Might Endanger the Pregnancy.
6. Even If You Don't Endanger the Pregnancy, If Something (God Forbid) Goes Wrong, You Will Forever Wonder If Your Exercising Caused It.
7. It's "Nine Months Up and Nine Months Down" in the Weight Department, No Matter What You Do (Give or Take a Few Months on the Downside).
8. Our Compulsion to Exercise When We Are Pregnant Is a Reflection of Our Inability to Surrender and Let Nature Run Its Course.

right, especially if you are newly pregnant. That's all right, but read this chapter anyway, if only for the enjoyment of trashing me afterward. You might just see things my way in the end.

1. You Will Be Too Tired

If the brain-numbing fatigue of early pregnancy has already struck you, then I don't need to go any further. You already know what it is like to sit on the side of your bed to tie your shoes and wake up two hours later. You have already made your peace with missing the rest of the season of *Lost* and have promised yourself you will catch up during summer reruns or buy the DVD. You have already humiliated yourself by falling asleep during a staff meeting and awakening so suddenly and awkwardly that you nearly fell off your chair and spilled a colleague's coffee.

If you are like the rest of us during our first pregnancies, you keep telling yourself that as soon as the first three months are over, you will get back to that class that promises to build your core. Like the rest of us, you will quietly be disturbed that you are such a weakling that you let a simple thing like pregnancy get in the way of your supreme fitness. You will be certain that other women—who *do* pregnancy *better* than you—are up at dawn for a quick five-mile sprint, instead of vomiting and then eating an entire pecan loaf for breakfast. Here is the news, Girlfriend: Even those jocky girls, the ones who were born with lean, muscular legs and lungs the size of all outdoors, tend to get soft and squishy during pregnancy. If they don't, then they are either in the microscopic minority, or they are depriving their babies and themselves of extremely valuable nutrition and rest. Besides, who wants to cuddle a mommy whose body is all sharp and pointy?

Here is a novel concept for the twenty-first century: If your body is tired, you should listen to it and rest. I am the last one to judge anyone poorly for being an activity addict in the nonpregnant state, but I sound the alarm when you have a human being growing in your abdomen. Think about it. From one little egg that you have had in your body since you were born, and one little sperm that your mate manufactured on the spur of the moment, you are expected to create an entire person. I'm talking arms, legs, heart, lungs, eyelashes, and your uncle Harry's big ears. If you don't think that can be tiring, then you are a pretty invincible woman, and not someone I yearn to spend much time with. The Girlfriends' recommendation is that you sleep whenever you possibly can during your pregnancy. You will not know this freedom again for several years.

2. You Won't Look like Yourself in the Harsh Gym Mirrors

At some point right around the three-month mark, you will probably begin to get your energy back. Not only will you get your old energy back, but you may actually feel *more* energetic than before you were pregnant. I call this the Wonder Woman Trimester. You probably aren't nauseous anymore. You may have regained your interest in sex (and then some, judging from the Girlfriends' reports). And you may consider taking up where you left off on the exercise regimen.

On your way out of your bedroom you catch a glimpse of yourself in your exercise attire. You do a double take. "Who is that squishy being, anyway?" Then you realize that the "squishy being" is you, and you run frantically to your bed to lie down before you faint. Even when you've sufficiently recovered to get to the gym, you may not be in the mood for the bad lighting that makes you look sallow, your eyes look baggy, and your cellulite visible *through* your Lycra pants.

Let's be brutally frank here. Everyone knows that skintight exercise clothes are primarily intended to show off our bodies. The manufacturers might insist that sleek Lycra is the most aerodynamic exercise fabric, and they might be right. But for the vast majority of us who haven't sprinted fifty meters since junior high school, aerodynamics are not all that crucial. We wear all that tight, stretchy stuff because we think we look good in it.

These sleek, little outfits take on a whole new identity when they are stuffed with pregnant breasts, pregnant bellies, pregnant thighs, and pregnant knees, and topped off by pregnant arms. If you don't take my word for it, rent yourself one of those home videos of exercise programs for pregnant women. I don't mean to be nasty, but the women in these videos look swollen and uncomfortable. And *those* are the women who looked good enough to volunteer to be on TV in their little, striped leotards in the first place! Those of us who would get dressed in absolute darkness to avoid having to inspect ourselves would rather have natural childbirth than have anyone see us in spandex at this point.

I have seen some die-hard pregnant women in the gym with their mate's T-shirt over their exercise clothes to camouflage things, and those who continue to wear their sexy workout clothes rolled under and over their curves, but I am one of those who would rather just sulk and stop exercising.

3. You Will Get Fat Anyway

I don't know about you, but I exercise in a constant effort to lose those last five pounds or to keep my derriere from resting on the backs of my thighs. Talk to me all you want to about endorphins, about restored energy, about cardiovascular fitness. I maintain that if we could all look like Kate Moss if we only lived on Red Bull and Marlboro Lights, all of the gyms in this country would close overnight, replaced by more 7-Elevens and ashtrays.

In pregnancy, the whole idea is to acknowledge that your body is now a baby-making machine. It needs to expand to allow for the growth of the baby. It also needs to fulfill its biological imperative to continue the species by adding stores of fat to make sure the baby doesn't starve even if the father fails to kill a boar for dinner one night. This is the opposite of what exercise fanatics are trying to do. Doesn't it make sense to you that you are making nature's job harder by following your quest for fat-burning activities? Why go through all that hard work when you won't look like Kate for at least another year, if ever?

I have noticed in those home exercise videos for pregnant women that a big deal is made of lifting light weights to keep the arms and upper body in shape. Since I have never seen "ripped" arms on a pregnant woman in my life, I have to assume they're doing these wussy little exercises in hopes that it won't take as long to get back in shape after the baby comes. I am not a physiologist, but my experience suggests that lifting two-pound weights or two cans of soup for twenty repetitions every day has nothing to do with how strong your arms will be after the baby is born. If lifting two soup cans is all it takes to keep a pregnant woman's muscles toned, why does the guy at my gym make me struggle with two fifteen-pound dumbbells when I am *not* pregnant? He certainly doesn't get paid by the pound!

4. Exercise Will Not Help You in Labor or Delivery in Any Way

The trendy logic goes something like this: Exercise builds strength and stamina. Labor and delivery require strength and stamina. Therefore, exercise must help during labor and delivery. Sounds reasonable, doesn't it? Well, we are here to tell you that it doesn't work that way. Labor is a series (seemingly endless) of *involuntary* muscle contractions. All of these involuntary contractions are supposed to result in the opening of the entrance to the uterus (the cervix) to a size of about ten centimeters. Then the mother is supposed to push the baby out of that opening.

You can do sit-ups from here till next Tuesday and they will not do one single thing to make your uterus stronger. Your uterus sits safely *behind* all of the muscles that are involved in the sit-up, and except for a Braxton Hicks contraction every now and then, it sits pretty quietly, minding its own business. If you think that you have come up with an exercise that can prepare your cervix to open quickly and on command, please let me know and we'll sell the patent to the Nautilus gym-equipment company and make a fortune. I'm just dying to know what it would look like.

You can also stretch, lunge, and lift weights all you want, and you will not become any more efficient at pushing. If you really want a preparatory exercise for pushing a baby out of your uterus, then have a lot of bowel movements, because they are probably as close to replicating the sensation as you are going to get. In fact, it could hurt you or your pregnancy if you consistently did exercises that forced you to do the bearing down and grunting that remind most of us of pushing. This tendency to hold your breath or grunt while exerting a particular muscle is called the Valsalvic maneuver, and most doctors agree that it isn't good for you or the baby. Evidently it unnaturally raises your blood pressure and momentarily slows the oxygen passing to the fetus.

I have watched many of my Girlfriends labor and deliver their babies, and one thing that never ceased to interest me was how irrelevant their fitness level was to the ease of their delivery. I have one Girlfriend who smoked cigarettes until the day she found out she was pregnant, then ate until the day she went into labor. She labored for three or four hours, then pushed the baby out in minutes. I have another Girlfriend who was a college track star and had maintained her fitness ever since. She labored for forty hours and never dilated past four centimeters. To my nonmedical eye, it almost looked as if the looser and less muscle-bound a woman was, the easier it was for the baby to get out. There is a certain poignancy here, because many Girlfriends work hard to stay physically fit and active and then have problematical deliveries, while many women who were petrified that they would never have the strength to make it through labor and delivery because their fitness regime consisted of walking briskly to the refrigerator are pleasantly surprised by their brilliant performance at getting that baby out. Once again, life illustrates its fundamental unfairness.

5. You Might Endanger the Pregnancy

Now I am purely speaking for myself. I may be the only woman on the face of the planet who has experienced this, and if I am, just indulge me for one moment, then forget I ever said anything. Early on in two of my four pregnancies, I tried to maintain my traditional exercise program of running and weight lifting, and two times I ended up with small tears where the placenta connects to the uterus. Apparently, lifting heavy weights applied too much pressure on my uterus. And two times I took to my bed crying and frightened for a day or two until the bleeding stopped. Who knows how much I endangered my babies? I was too terrified to ask my doctor *that* question—or more to the point, too terrified to hear his answer. I do know, however, that my doctor did a number of ultrasounds to monitor the healing, and that he was relieved when he saw no more blood pooling up in there, so I guess he had been somewhat concerned, too.

A point could be made that I was exercising too strenuously, and that I should have modified my exercise routine rather than ended it. Most of the current wisdom says that a pregnant woman can continue exercising to her full capacity, but that she should not take up *new* or *more difficult* regimens after becoming pregnant. To be completely candid with you, I did not know how to exercise moderately. If I wasn't working out to achieve strength or to stay trim, I would just as soon skip the whole thing. Since the stakes were so high, I wasn't willing to gamble with how much was too much. And since there comes a point when exercising lightly becomes a waste of time, I just gave the whole thing up.

6. Even If You Don't Endanger the Pregnancy, If Something (God Forbid) Goes Wrong, You Will Forever Wonder If Your Exercising Caused It

When we become pregnant, we become obsessed about taking care of the pregnancy. We invest so much physical and emotional nurturing because we start to love that baby when it is no bigger than a lima bean. Tragically, not all pregnancies result in the delivery of a healthy baby. The most common threat to a successful pregnancy is miscarriage. It happens more often than you might think; estimates say about 10 percent of all known pregnancies end in miscarriage, and more if the mother is older or very young. The vast majority of miscarriages occur during the first three months of pregnancy. It is widely believed that about half of all miscarriages occur because the fetus was not normal. Thus comes the most common, and least comforting, comment that a woman who has just miscarried will receive: "Don't worry, dear. This is just nature's way of weeding out the imperfect ones."

It is also widely believed that exercise, stress, intercourse, and jumping off a chair will *not* cause miscarriage. So I guess that big scene when Rhett pushes Scarlett down the stairs and she loses their baby is biologically inaccurate. It is definitely true that when you are seventeen and have missed your period, all of the jumping, douching, and praying in the world won't seem to do anything to interrupt a pregnancy. I don't know, however, if it is completely true in women who, like me, had a bleeding episode or used fertility drugs to get pregnant. If frequent exercise and intercourse have no bearing whatsoever on miscarriage, then why do so many good doctors prescribe "full pelvic rest" (no sex) when the woman seems at risk for miscarriage?

My big question is, how do you know you are having a risky pregnancy until you push yourself and something goes wrong, such as when I started bleeding after bench-pressing? What if I'd lost that baby? My doctor could have sworn on his own children (although I doubt he would have) that my pumping iron and the loss of the baby were purely coincidental, but I would never totally have believed him. I find the mantle of guilt easy to don, and just as I won't stand within three feet of working microwaves when I am pregnant (I know, this is inconsistent with my cavalier attitude about hair coloring, but indulge me) just in case all the scientific evidence is wrong and they *are* dangerous, I won't exercise either, just in case. Nine (ten) months, give or take a few weeks for recovery, is not really very long to give up strenuous exercise if it can help you maintain a clear conscience. Besides, it could be a well-deserved vacation.

7. It's "Nine Months Up and Nine Months Down" in the Weight Department, No Matter What You Do (Give or Take a Few Months on the Downside).

Some of you will hate me for saying this, and some of you will be grateful and relieved. It usually breaks down like this: Those of you who are newly pregnant will hate me for telling you that it will take so long to get your old self back, because, in essence, I am telling you to be patient with your imperfect figure for almost a year and a half. On the other hand, those of you who have recently given birth will be grateful and relieved, because you will realize that you are not alone in your inability to wear your favorite clothes four months after the baby is born. (Please don't start in with me about your friend who wore her jeans home from the hospital. I know that there are miracles, but I think it is safer not to count on their happening to us mortals. If it makes you feel any better, speculate about the eating disorders they may secretly be harboring.)

When the baby is born, assuming it is of average size, you will lose about ten or twelve pounds during and shortly after the delivery. If you are like my Girlfriend Monique, you will then retain water so badly that you will regain about five water pounds within twenty-four hours. After you pee and sweat away another five to seven pounds over the next week, you will be left with at least ten to fifteen pounds that you didn't have before pregnancy. Or, if you are like my Girlfriend Lisa, you will have forty unfamiliar pounds upholstering your little bones.

There is a biological reason for this extra weight. Food is the biggest and most obvious one. But the more pertinent question might be, Why are you so much hungrier when you are pregnant and nursing? One answer might be that you need to bulk up to sustain this baby inside you and to feed it when it is born. You might also need extra food for a while postpartum to help your body regain its strength after pregnancy and delivery, neither of which is a day at the beach. My big gripe is that we get so hung up on the F-word (as in *Fat*) that we fail to understand that some greater wisdom is governing our weight gain and loss.

As an experiment, I started working to lose weight when my fourth child was six weeks old. Usually it had been my style to take it easy until four to six months postpartum, but after being pregnant or nursing for nearly seven years without much of a break, I decided to wean the baby and aggressively try to reclaim my former self. I exercised like a lunatic.

No matter how hard you are used to exercising, I did it harder and longer. I ran, mountain-hiked, or StairMastered a minimum of sixty minutes, and more frequently ninety minutes, a day, at least five days a week. I lifted weights with a trainer who felt that repetitions had to be so intense that you saw stars and whimpered during the workout. And, yes, I did lose weight pretty quickly. But I *did not* get my old figure back until my baby was more than nine months old.

Then there is my Girlfriend Amy, who was so busy with her baby and traveling because of her husband's work that she never really exercised until the baby was nearly a year old. *And she, too, had her old figure back at about nine months postpartum.* Something magical just seems to happen around that time that makes your body ready to let go of the fat it has been hiding under your arms, between your legs, and around your middle. As long as you are no longer eating like a pregnant or nursing woman, you will drop the weight. An exception, of course, is if you are still nursing after nine months. People will tell you that nursing burns up a lot of calories, and it does, but it also encourages your body to hold on to an extra five to ten pounds to keep that milk factory in operation. Heck, your breasts alone are probably five pounds heavier than they ever were before. So you should not expect to drop down to your sleek former self until you have stopped nursing entirely.

Another change in your figure on which exercising has absolutely no effect is the loosening of your ligaments. For you to pass that baby out between your hips, your pelvic bones have to widen and separate. This means that, even if the scale says you have lost all of your weight, you may still not be able to fit into your old pants. Here, too, it is just a matter of time. After about nine months, or even up to a year, you will find your bones going back to where they used to be.

It would be a good idea if women (*and their doctors*) stopped thinking that the time required for recovery from pregnancy and delivery is six weeks. That is absolute bullshit, and it really does a disservice to women to lead them into believing something is wrong with them if they are not back to their old selves a month and a half after creating and birthing a complete human being. You won't feel the same, and you shouldn't expect to *look* the same, that quickly. If nature didn't keep you a "little bit pregnant" until your baby was old enough to eat something other than mother's milk, you might be tempted to wander off and get pregnant again. See, it's not you, it's *nature* that makes you have to wear maternity jeans five months after the baby is born!

8. Our Compulsion to Exercise When We Are Pregnant Is a Reflection of Our Inability to Surrender and Let Nature Run Its Course

"SURRENDER, DOROTHY!"

Get ready now: I am climbing onto my soapbox for this one, because it is the foundation for the philosophy of this entire book. The greatest lesson in life, and particularly in pregnancy, is to BE NICE TO YOURSELF. It is time to *really* understand that your body was intended for more than just being a vehicle through which you amuse yourself, promote yourself, or abuse yourself. It is designed to gestate a baby. Nature has wisely put you on automatic pilot because she knows that, if left to your own devices, you might mess the whole thing up. All you have to do is behave moderately and surrender; nature will do the rest. Try as you might, you don't control whether you will have a boy or a girl (unless you're a subscriber to the gender-selection technology that's out there), you don't control when the baby will be born (unless you induce labor), and you have absolutely no control over your body. And really, when you come to think of it, why should you? You don't know anything about making babies. If having a baby required a preparatory degree, the species would have died out eons ago.

My observation is that a lot of my Girlfriends who continue to exercise rigorously during pregnancy are frantically trying to take back control of a life that they think is spinning out on them. Their bodies are distorting in more ways than they ever imagined, their emotions seem out of control, and they are frightened of giving birth and becoming a parent. No one can blame you for trying to get a grip on things by acting as if nothing strange were happening. I remember how people used to try that when they experimented with LSD in the seventies. They just told themselves to act "normal" to try to keep from freaking out. The truth is, it didn't work then, and it doesn't work now. You can get out your *Yoga Booty Ballet* videotape every day, and it won't make you any more in charge of what is going on with your body. You can Tony Little your way through pregnancy, but if you think that you are guaranteeing yourself a more "perfect" pregnancy, you are deluding yourself. If, however, you are continuing to exercise (and ignoring *The Girlfriends' Guide*) because it makes you feel good and you enjoy it, then knock yourself out—within reason.

Exceptions to My Tirade

There. Now that I have made my basic points about exercising, I want to back off in a couple of areas. First, there are two benefits to some forms of *moderate* exercise that I have neglected to mention, and those are *relaxation* and *flexibility*. You might want to dance, swim (if you are brave enough to put on a bathing suit), do yoga, or (my personal favorite) walk. These activities oxygenate your blood and help get the kinks out without making you overheated or exhausted. As I've mentioned, pregnancy can have its stressful moments, and getting "out of your head" in some physical way can be helpful.

Pregnancy is also quite demanding on your body and can lead to all sorts of aches and pains. My Girlfriend Patti, who wasn't keen on exercising for its own sake during pregnancy, took it up in her third pregnancy with a certified trainer to help ease the soreness in her sciatic nerve (which runs from your spine all the way down the back of your leg and can become inflamed during pregnancy). She still gained a respectable Girlfriend's amount of weight (at least thirty-five pounds), but her back felt better.

The best advice I can give you if you are going to continue with your exercise program is to move it outdoors whenever possible. First of all, there are fewer mirrors outdoors, and second, there are fewer gym odors outdoors (and we all know what havoc foul odors can wreak on a nauseous pregnant woman!).

A lot of pregnant women really enjoy swimming. About halfway through your pregnancy you will begin to realize the appeal of buoyancy. My Girlfriends found swimming a tremendous relief because it provided a respite from lugging all that weight around. I, too, loved that buoyancy, but I chose to experience it in my bubbly bathtub, not in the local YMCA pool.

Walking is also great because you get your circulation moving and get a chance to think at the same time. One of the best things about walking is its value during labor: It gets that baby pressing down on the cervix and can help move your dilation along. But more about that later.

Kegels—the Most Important Exercises You Can Do

Kegels are a series of exercises that are designed to strengthen an area known as your pelvic floor. I have absolutely no idea where my pelvic floor is, but I do know that committing to a regimen of Kegels can help with such things as bladder control and sexual enjoyment after pregnancy. You might need to tighten up that pelvic floor because it gets mighty stretched out during a vaginal delivery (which might explain the trend toward scheduled C-sections I'm noticing).

One of the deepest, darkest secrets about pregnancy is the amount of stretching and loosening your vagina and surrounding tissues will endure. It is a secret because women are embarrassed by the legacies of this wear and tear, which are conditions known as incontinence and flaccidity. In other words, a woman who has vaginally delivered a baby or two might find that she pees a little when she sneezes or jumps, and jogging can be a real bladder breaker. Flaccidity refers to a weakening of the vaginal muscles that makes it harder *for your partner* to reach orgasm because the muscles aren't "gripping" his penis with their former strength. I think it is pretty easy to understand why most mothers don't talk about their pelvic floor. Who wants to say that she wets her pants and has moved from a regular to a supersize Tampax—and that even *that* slips out when she sneezes? The feminine mystique stands to take a real beating here.

I can just hear the groaning going on now and the exclamations of disbelief. But if your Girlfriends don't tell you, then how can we help you avoid or cure the problem? If what I am saying were not true, why are the majority of obstetricians so willing to "take a couple of extra stitches" when they repair your episiotomy to "tighten things up a bit down there"? They are certainly not trying to sew your vagina *closed*!

Here's how you learn how to do your Kegels: You sit on the toilet with your legs apart and stop and start the flow of urine several times. Whatever muscles you are using to stop the flow of urine are the muscles that you use to do Kegels. In fact, while you are learning your Kegel fitness program, you should practice this "stutter peeing" whenever you use the toilet. Once you have gotten stronger and more familiar with the sensation, you can move on to the party-tricks section. It is the Girlfriends' experience that "stutter peeing" alone is not rigorous enough to make much of an improvement in your vaginal muscles; what you are looking for is strength and endurance.

Therefore, the next Kegel exercise you should master is the tightening-and-holding technique. Try this: The next time you are sitting in your car at a red light, see if you can keep those vaginal muscles tight without stopping until the light turns green. Or, if you are watching television, see if you can stay "flexed" throughout an entire commercial. Just don't forget to keep breathing. You will know if you are doing the tightening-and-holding maneuver correctly if you begin to feel anxious and uncomfortable. Honest, when this exercise is done correctly, my Girlfriends Amy and Shannon and I agree that it makes you feel slightly nervous inside. You can even feel light-headed. It's like orgasm without the O.

As you near the end of your pregnancy, you may find Kegels harder to do. This is because all of the soft tissue in and around your vagina starts to swell as the baby puts more pressure down there. Don't worry if you feel as if your Kegels are completely ineffective—just keep doing them. As soon as the baby is born, start up again and do them whenever you think about it for the rest of your life. You will thank me for sharing this, and your partner (or any future sex partner) will thank me, too.

9
Sex and Pregnancy

YOU'RE PREGNANT, RIGHT? Clearly you're familiar with the fundamentals of sex, right? After all, if you didn't know something about the birds and the bees, you wouldn't be in this predicament in the first place. (On the other hand, if you knew more about sex, maybe you *wouldn't* be in this predicament!) If you're feeling a little smug right now, you will only labor (pun intended) under that delusion for a short time—because most pregnant women quickly realize that pregnant sex and regular sex are two *very* different things. We can all agree that, under normal circumstances, our sexuality involves our bodies and our minds. In fact, really good sex is almost always more emotional than physical, especially for the Girlfriends.

It is clearly no news flash that a pregnant woman's body is radically changing and that this change is matched twist for turn by her emotional changes. These changes will most definitely affect how you feel about sex, and how your mate feels about it, too. And while not everyone feels the same about pregnant sex, everyone can be put into one of two different categories: those who love it more during pregnancy and those who love it less. And because Mother Nature is nothing if not fun, you and your mate may not be in the same category at the same time.

Your body is already different, and if you are anything like me, it will continue to change until it takes on cartoonlike proportions. *Bountiful* is the operative word here, Girlfriends: bountiful booty, bountiful breasts, bountiful belly, and usually bountiful arms, thighs, and face. In fact, one of the greatest sexual challenges is just figuring out how to negotiate the hills and valleys of the pregnant body to reach the mother lode, so to speak. How you feel physically and emotionally in this psycho body will deeply affect your sexuality. And if you think it's a trip for you, wait until I tell you about some of the reactions of your partners. Some of them are aroused by all this bounty, and some of them are terrified by it. You may already have your suspicions as to which category your mate will perch in.

The other operative word here is *hormonal*. The progesterone poisoning that we discussed in chapter 4 has an emotional component, as well. Not only must you cope with the emotional whiplash of going from a nonpregnant to a pregnant state, your libido is also going haywire. One minute you might feel as lusty and sexy as Jessica Rabbit, and the next you feel as ungainly as Baby Huey. Then at times you are so uninterested in sex that you threaten mayhem to anyone who approaches you (continuing on a theme, think Tasmanian Devil for this cartoon analogy). Unless you do something quite overt, such as change colors with your moods, your partner might never know who is lying in wait for him (or her). My poor husband tried to avoid making any eye contact with me until he was able to determine if I was Rational Vicki or Feral Vicki.

As if you don't already have your hands full, what with trying to deal with your physical and emotional changes as a pregnant woman, nature really complicates matters by asking you to deal with your hapless partner's, as well. If nurturing someone else through this trying time while trying to survive it yourself seems like an overwhelming task, do what Girlfriends have been doing for years: Ignore your partner and concentrate on yourself. Remember, without you, this pregnancy is a bust. Without your mate, it's just another sad statistic. Harsh, but true.

And Baby Makes Three

You may not even look pregnant yet, but still, it is no longer just the two of you in bed. Both you and your mate are keenly aware that someone else is there with you. Even if the baby is only the size of a raisin, its existence has a profound effect on how both parents view sex. When guys fantasize about a ménage à trois, this probably isn't what they had in mind. This little observer, your baby, might make you or your mate feel inhibited in the way you express yourself sexually, especially in the beginning. If you feel this, don't worry—eventually pure horniness will be enough to get both of you over the hump, so to speak. If it doesn't, relax and know that you are not the first two people to have had your sex life destroyed by parenthood; it just hits some of us earlier rather than later. Just wait until you have two or three kids running in and out of your bedroom, or even sleeping in your bed, to see the utter devastation of some active sex lives. If you feel too self-conscious to talk dirty and yell because of a tiny little fetus, you'll have a hell of a challenge being fully present during the deed when you have a six-year-old hiding under your bed or are including your in-laws in your intimacy with your cell phone's unexpected conference-call capabilities.

Sex like Mom and Dad Used to Have

All of a sudden, you and your mate have been transformed by this new pregnancy from two people with the spiritual inner life of the kids from the *OC* into *Somebody's Parents*. How terrifying is that? The responsibilities of parenthood can be so frightening that it is often the breeding ground for some profound sexual changes during pregnancy. The very personality traits that attracted you in the first place may seem reprehensible in a potential coparent.

My Girlfriend Dina's husband, who loved her habit of walking around the house in a short nightie with no panties on before she got pregnant, immediately insisted that she start wearing *proper* pj's with tops and bottoms after she got pregnant. He found the sexual come-on that had so delighted him before to be completely inappropriate for the mother of his child. My Girlfriend Tory, married to a musician (and we all know how *those* guys are), had lots and lots of red-hot monkey sex with him before pregnancy, then found his late nights out and his partying with the boys to be a real drag when she got pregnant. Before long, his tattooed body stopped turning her on, and she found herself yearning to be with any man, gay or straight, who appeared in Ralph Lauren or J.Crew catalogs— she even confessed in a moment of weakness to going into a Brooks Brothers to admire the silk ties.

One of the most difficult emotional conflicts that couples encounter in their pregnant sex life is that we all secretly harbor the belief that our parents never really *did it,* or at least not as nastily as we did. We are also, consciously or subconsciously, loathe to imagine the particulars, if they did. If your mate begins to have the same expectations about you that he learned from his mother, Girlfriend, you may find yourself with little more to do at night than daydream about your vibrator and wonder if he'd hear it if you plugged it in, in the bathroom. I remember that when my guy first fell for me, I wore skinny, white jeans tucked into boots and had long, red fingernails. When he got serious enough to want to marry me and start a family, he told me he'd really appreciate it if I'd lose the nails and the boots. But hear me on this point: When I want to stir up some action today, I go right to my manicurist for a set of acrylics and pull out my "fuck me" boots (you Girlfriends know what I'm talkin' about!).

You've all heard of the madonna (not that Madonna!)/whore complex, where the guy wants fun, party sex with "whores," but will only accept a "madonna" as the mother of his child. Rumor has it that Elvis never touched Priscilla again after she got pregnant with Lisa Marie. (At least that's what Priscilla maintained later to justify sleeping with her karate teacher.) Psychoanalysts have mined this territory of the emotional life of men ad nauseam, and I certainly can't add anything to their work. The only advice the Girlfriends have is this: If you think you are married to an Elvis, take it in stride and play against type. If your mate thinks of you as the Virgin Mother now that you are pregnant, you owe it to both of you to occasionally throw to the back of the closet all the sundresses and baby-doll prints that send your mother and her friends into rapture and look for something black with lots of cleavage and stilettos to match. Do whatever it takes to remind him that you are not yet his or anyone else's mother and are so irresistible that he remembers why he knocked you up in the first place.

"There's Only Room for One of Us in There"

Another emotional issue for many guys is the popular worry that, by having intercourse with you, they will inadvertently harm the baby. I just love this one! From what I can gather in my conversations with prospective fathers, their thinking seems to go something like this: If the tiny little baby is accidentally in the path of the BIG, STRONG, THROBBING BATTERING RAM that is his, it might be killed, or at least left defective. Isn't that so cute, you could just grab his ram and squeeze it off right now? It's just like a man to overestimate both the size and penetration of his member. I have even heard some men suggest that they could *feel* the pregnancy with the tip of their penis during rigorous sex. One can't help but marvel at the confidence (or folly) that such a comment implies. It's rather like a woman saying that her sweet stuff can pull him in and hold him against his will.

It would take a *very* long penis with extraordinary sensitivity to accomplish what these guys are fretting about. I've *dreamed* about a guy like that.

All kidding aside, I have heard of several men who were so freaked-out by this battering-ram concept that they couldn't get it up for intercourse with their pregnant mate. Now, for those Girlfriends who are indifferent to sex at this time in their life, this may sound like a cloud with a sterling-silver lining, but don't get out the polish just yet. On second thought, DO, because there's a great pun here: Just because a guy isn't up for intercourse doesn't mean he doesn't want to know some satisfaction, Girlfriend. We all know that oral sex is always welcome and maybe never more than now, and you may have a lot of "polishing" asked of you. To my way of thinking, this is just one more chore for Mommy, and we can decline on the grounds of heartburn or an uncontrollable gag reflex (my personal fave).

As funny as this battering-ram story is, there is some truth to it, according to many of my Girlfriends. Several of them told me that they didn't enjoy energetic intercourse as much as before because their partner's rams *were* slightly painful or distressing because they reached the cervix, which was sensitive. The *cervix,* mind you, not the baby in the *uterus.* If you have a special reason, rational or not, to fear miscarriage, you might want to skip intercourse for a while and just enjoy the related delicacies until you and/or your doctor say it's safe. It's good to know that, particularly in the last stages of pregnancy, semen contains a chemical that can help bring on the dilation of the cervix in preparation for the baby's birth. That information may make you cautious now, but when your due date has come and gone, you'll be begging for some of that stuff.

The Genie Is Out of the Bottle

One pleasant emotional benefit of pregnant sex is that there is no longer any need to worry about getting pregnant. I know that sounds like nonsense, but even if you were really intending to get pregnant, you might still have felt some ambivalence. Once conception has occurred, however, you will relax and stop second-guessing yourself—especially if you have learned your Surrender Lesson from earlier in this *Girlfriends' Guide.* After fifteen years of worrying about my birth control failing me, it was such a relief not to have to give it a thought. The barn door had been left open, the cow had escaped, and now I could leave the door open and have a fine old time swinging on it. If you relied on birth control methods that required goopy spermicides or condoms or other slippery stuff, you and yours are in for a treat.

Because everyone is entitled (encouraged!) to march to the beat of his or her own drummer, I feel obligated to mention those people who say they find the absence of the fear of pregnancy to have a *dampening* effect. These are the thrill seekers, the drama junkies, the people who get a little high when the stakes are, too. Lots of these people are guys who like extreme sports, where death is a possibility and serious harm is a given. But just as many are girls: the ones who like a guy who doesn't always call when he says he will, or who has strange text messages from people named "hornybaby" or "moan4me." These are the people who were turned on by the sexual Russian roulette of wondering each time if they'd escaped pregnancy. Now that they are caught, they need a moment to figure out the next obvious risk, to keep the adrenaline flowing. I have a suggestion: how about getting health insurance in your name and your mate's, and trying to give the baby a mom and a dad? Just a crazy thought . . .

Just as I know plenty of drama junkies, I know an equal number of people, usually women, who think the conception of a baby is the only real reason to have sex in the first place. Sure, it's fun and something to do on a Friday night, but that's just the appetizer before the entrée: reproduction. When these people (Girlfriends) discover they are pregnant, they find any sexual overtures from their mate inconvenient at best, and at worst, well, redundant. To them, pregnancy means nine (ten) months of not having to shave their legs. I call this the Precious Vessel approach toward gestation; these gals do not want to be messed with in any physical way, besides foot massages and shoulder rubs, until after the baby arrives and is weaned. Unfortunately, many of these Girlfriends are hooked up with men who find this as good a time as any to consider an affair.

If the affair stuff is actually a relief to you, then bless you and yours. I guess you could say that everyone is getting his or her needs met. But if it's driving a stake of terror into you, this might be the time to smile pretty and dust off those faking-orgasm skills.

The Potent Seed and the Fertile Soil

Another positive emotional reaction to the news that you are pregnant is the booster shot to a couple's sense of potency and fecundity. Rare is the man who fails to puff up his chest with pride when told he has impregnated his woman. Men just love to know that the howitzer is in good working order and that it's shooting live ammo. As long as there have been babies, there have been men and women who feel such pride that it seems as if they hold the patent on the process. My Girlfriend Taylor got so earth-mothery and sensual when she learned she was pregnant that visiting her at her home meant being greeted by Buddhist wind chimes and world music. She always had some foul herbal tea brewing that she delighted in drinking over ice with a cinnamon stick. Being in her proximity started to feel like being a voyeur to her sexual witchcraft, and I couldn't take it for long, but I was always in awe of her and her luxuriant sexual satisfaction. If her partner came home when I was there, I would bolt for the door because he would enter like Zeus uniting with Hera and I felt like a mortal who could not witness such things. They were gods on Mount Olympus, delighting over their coupling and eager to plow those mighty fields again and again. I was kind of grossed out, but that's just me.

Multiple Personality Disorder, Anyone?

The thing that amazed my Girlfriends and me about the emotional life of pregnant women, particularly where sex was concerned, was the intensity of all the emotions you feel and the rapidity with which they change. You may spend the entire day fantasizing about wild animal sex with your partner, to the point where you chew off all your fingernails waiting for him to meet you at home. Then, when he finally arrives and starts going through the mail instead of studying the ultrasound photos that you just got, *without him,* at your morning appointment and have lovingly placed on the front door, you start screaming that this is one more undeniable sign that he is indifferent to you and the baby. By the time he has calmed you down and you go whimpering into the bathroom to refresh yourself and consider whether you're still horny, you've fallen asleep in the tub and he's pulling you out before you drown.

It's as if your emotional engine is stuck at fourth gear and running full throttle all the time. You don't build up to a feeling so much as arrive at it going ninety miles an hour. Worse yet, your brakes are no good and you're not sure if the power steering works. Just as a pregnant woman is never just a *little bit* hungry, she is never just *mildly interested* in sex and she doesn't get just a *tad impatient* with his inability to anticipate and react properly to her moods. She is a savage and she will not be denied!

According to my unscientific survey for this *Girlfriends' Guide,* the split is about sixty-forty between pregnant women who become more sexual and those who become almost completely uninterested. Of course, if you're a guy, you won't believe me, but what else is new? We Girlfriends can play the game, and we do so when it suits us. You will probably never know what we're thinking when we're doing that. Anyway, back to the matter at hand. My Girlfriend Tracy felt constantly aroused while pregnant, and the father of her baby was more than happy to oblige her appetites. Thinking back on it, however, Tracy was what I now call a Geisha Wife: She was such a man-pleaser that she would have made herself feel hot even if her feet were packed in ice. Then there was my Girlfriend Tawny, who was completely distracted by her pregnancy and didn't much notice if she was having sex or not; but because her mate was always turned on by her, they kept it pretty active. To this day, I don't know if she recalls any of it. As for me, I vividly recall stalking my husband for sexual fulfillment as soon as my morning sickness passed. I would linger near the front door or surprise him in the garage. Funny, now that I think of it, he always had a slightly fearful expression in those days. And he was mighty jumpy, too.

Mr. Sandman, Bring Me a Dream . . .

By the second trimester of my pregnancies, I thought about sex almost constantly. And when I wasn't thinking about it, I was dreaming about it. Let me tell you, these dreams were absolutely fantastic. The erotic fantasy life I enjoyed during REM sleep convinced me that progesterone is a psychedelic. I'm not just talking about your ordinary sex dream where you and Brad Pitt are on a train together, entering a tunnel. I'm talking about really lifelike dreams where you're not only watching yourself have sex, but you're FEELING IT and it's not just with movie idols, old boyfriends, or you own partner, but with just about *any* man (or woman!) you saw that day. For me, that could mean my UPS guy, the manager at Whole Foods, or even friends of my husband's. Taste and propriety were no concerns of my somnolent life. (Although I did feel icky when my minister showed up in one of my dreams with a lean and hungry look on his face. I confess that I still find a robe and collar to be a turn-on, which is weird with all the priestly pedophilia that's come out since then.) David Letterman also came to me several times in my dreams. Sure, he might seem chilly and distant to you, but when I fell asleep to his show night after night, I thawed him out just fine. I'm just glad I never watched *The O'Reilly Factor* on Fox at that time of night.

While the dreams were pretty great, I still haven't told you the best part, and for this I'm willing to swear on a stack of Dave's Top Ten Lists: I FREQUENTLY EXPERIENCED FULL AND ACTUAL PHYSICAL ORGASM IN THESE DREAMS. On my honor as a Girlfriend. And I've learned I'm not the only one who was blessed with this divine ability; other Girlfriends have shyly come forward with similar tales. The first time it happened to me, I woke up thinking there had been an earthquake (after all, I live in California). It was such a jolt that I scared my dog, Laika, who was lying beside my bed. Best of all, it wasn't completely over yet, so I knew that this baby was the real thing. It wasn't a *dream* about an orgasm, it *was* an orgasm and I was still feeling it! Aren't you happy for me, Girlfriends? I woke up shuddering and then wanting a cigarette, all with no hands and no assistance. God, I miss that. Actually, I usually woke up wanting more, and I would shake my husband awake and rub up against him in hopes of helping him catch up with me.

When I shared this secret with a friend, a man, over a giddy lunch, the idea for this book was born. He slapped the table and got so excited that he called a literary agent right there from the restaurant and said, "Bookie, you are never going to believe what Vicki Iovine just told me about her pregnant dreams!" The rest is a dream of a different sort, but I digress.

Ready, Willing, and Able

Those women who are not completely put off by sex while pregnant will probably find they are much *more* interested now. More interested than they've been since those make-out sessions in steamy cars and Mile High Club encounters with total strangers. One of the most logical explanations for a pregnant woman's increased lust is her copious hormonal surges and the engorgement of her sexual organs. The organs are more easily stimulated (if we're in the right head space), and the owners of those organs follow their lead. When you're pregnant, your labia, like your nipples, not only become darker in color and more sensitive—they get progressively more engorged with blood. WAIT, I need a drink of water before I can continue with this. . . . Isn't this fun?

OK, back to what I was saying. This engorgement is like what happens when you are sexually aroused. If you don't believe us, Girlfriend, get yourself a hand mirror and check for yourself. Kind of gives a new meaning to the phrase *power walking,* doesn't it?

The Titty Fairy

My Girlfriend Sondra's husband calls the rapid growth spurt of a pregnant woman's breasts the arrival of the Titty Fairy. He hit on an apt metaphor because their metamorphosis seemed to happen almost overnight. After your first missed period you will probably notice some swelling and soreness, but the breasts still seem familiarly premenstrual. No big deal. But in about another month, you will wake one morning to find that they have really become bigger, to the point where your bras no longer fit and you have cleavage where you've never had it before. We Girlfriends have all noticed that this change in size and, well, *ripeness* seems to happen suddenly and dramatically, especially in this surreal state of being. And then our breasts continued to grow for the rest of the first trimester. For those of us who don't normally have much to begin with, this is the gift that keeps on giving. Eventually, our bustline is outpaced by our bellies and their ripeness is less dramatic than before, but until then, it's like a piñata party and we're the ones filled with candy.

Early in your pregnancy, especially if this is your first, you will have two or three months when the rest of your body looks fairly normal but your breasts are heavy and full, just like the heaving ones they describe in romance novels. I have yet to hear of a man who wasn't deeply moved by this development (yeah, I know, another pun). More important, I have yet to hear of a Girlfriend who wasn't equally moved.

As we have discussed, at this point your breasts will be particularly sensitive. You might want to point this biological fact out to your mate, since his enthusiastic delight in them might make you want to holler in pain. After your appreciative partner has been properly sensitized to the need for a light touch, you may actually find this breast sensitivity to be erotic; some of my Girlfriends have reported being able to climax through breast stimulation alone. But a word of warning: As you get near your delivery date, breast stimulation can bring on or intensify labor. Yes, it's true: Nipple-twisting is actually recommended by your granola pregnancy books as an organic oxytocin stimulator. Oxytocin is the natural chemical that induces labor. Mother Nature is a genius, isn't she? Your doctor may give you the pharmaceutical equivalent, pitocin, to speed up your labor when the time comes. Anyway, accept this as cautionary intelligence and talk to your doctor about it if you have any concerns about premature labor or miscarriage. Conversely, if your due date has come and gone and you're impatiently awaiting your baby's arrival, stimulate and twist to your heart's content. The side benefit of all this breast handling is that it toughens up your nipples in preparation for nursing.

By the way, in case you are not reading this *Girlfriends' Guide* in chapter order, I will take the opportunity again to tell you to rock on with your big breasts! In fact, consider getting some artful pregnancy nudes taken, because after you have finished gestating and nursing, your twins will be much smaller and far less perky. If this is news to you, I am sorry—but if your Girlfriends won't tell you the truth, who will? Besides, if and when you get pregnant again, the piñata party begins again.

Oral Sex

Oral sex is almost always fun, and it should continue to be so during pregnancy, especially when intercourse is problematical. But you should know about a few physiological changes so that you and your partner can be prepared. For example, the engorgement of your sexual organs and their change in color might not be noticeable to your mate during intercourse, but during oral sex the changes really are *in his face.* It would probably be a good idea to mention this casually before he notices them, because surprise is not always an aphrodisiac.

You would be very considerate if you also prepared him for the change in your *flavor* down there, if he hasn't already tasted it for himself. There is some scientific explanation for this, having to do with the uterine lining going from alkaline to acidic, or vice versa, and it's completely normal. I didn't know a thing about this until my Girlfriend Susie, who has three kids now, told me that her husband could always tell she was pregnant even before she suspected it herself by his discriminating taste. Talk about a home pregnancy test.

Bigger and Bigger and BIGGER!

One thing that always seemed unfair to me was that as I grew increasingly interested in sex, I also just plain grew. Loving as my husband is, I knew there came a point when having sex with me was more a mercy mission than an act of passion—not that I cared at the time. Look, everyone is different, but a significant number of men are not really turned on by partners who weigh more than they do (and eat twice as much as they do).

As I have mentioned, when I was pregnant with my second child, I had some spotting in my third month. My doctor advised that I forgo intercourse for four to six weeks. Naturally, I opted to forgo it for seven weeks, just to be safe. When I was first "benched," I was still reasonably trim and sexy, but by the time I felt it was safe to have sex again, I had unknowingly begun to resemble a character from *Fantasia.* Naively, I parked our first-born with my Girlfriend and began my preparations for the big reunion. I washed and hot-rolled my hair, put on enough makeup to appear in the chorus of *Hairspray,* and slipped into (OK, *tugged on*) a silk camisole and matching panties. Well, I might as well have opened a parasol and walked the high wire, for how much I looked like the ballerina hippos in the Disney classic. My husband was so struck by the sight that his normal sense of self-preservation escaped him and he laughed uncontrollably at me. His funny bone was so deeply and genuinely struck that he was willing to risk his life to indulge it. He still gets a tear in his eye when he remembers it.

My experience is not universal, however; some men just love their women fat and sassy and are totally turned on by their big, beautiful baby mamas. My Girlfriend Shannon tells me that, as far as her mate was concerned, the bigger she was, the better he liked her. He would whoop and holler during sex with her, just like a cowboy on his bronco. Her gigantic breasts and big booty were as inviting as any living thing could be. He particularly enjoyed talking nasty to her during sex because it felt scandalous to him to talk that way to a mother.

No More Missionary Style

During the first few months of pregnancy, almost any sexual position works. The only real hazards are those ever-sensitive breasts we've talked about; they often can't bear the pressure of a man lying on them. Later, as the belly grows, having sex can be like playing Twister, it becomes so challenging to accommodate the bumps, curves, and sensitive spots. You will eventually discover two disagreeable things about the old man-on-top, woman-on-her-back missionary style: First, lying flat on your back forces the baby to rest on one of your major arteries, thereby cutting off your circulation and making you feel faint. Second, the full belly between you and your partner can make frontal penetration nearly impossible, unless your partner has a twenty-four-inch penis, in which case he should consider charging stud fees.

Sometime in the middle of the pregnancy, a lot of couples move on to the position quaintly known as doggy style. This is where the woman is on her hands and knees and the man is behind her. Most of my Girlfriends agree that this position can allow the husband to penetrate too deeply, so if it is not practiced with restraint, it can hurt. A popular variation on that theme is one we call spoons, and we Girlfriends recommend it whole-heartedly. In this position the man and woman lie on their sides, facing the same direction. It's cuddly, it gives a lot of skin-to-skin sensation, *and* you can hold a pillow between your knees and hips for support if you want to. (More about the Girlfriends' affection for their pillows later in this *Girlfriends' Guide*.)

Good ol' Sexy Shannon shared with me a position that I have found pure genius. It was so good, in fact, that I mentioned it to Maryann the other day and now she's a convert, too. Shannon and her partner loved having sex in their bathroom. In fact, if the legend is true, one of her kids was conceived in that sacred room. She would lean over the sink and he could come up behind her. The positioning was just right to admire their reflections in the mirror and do the deed. As an added bonus the sink and counter came up to just the right height to hide her biggest parts and highlight the Girls to their best advantage. Hey, if you can brush your teeth at the same time, there's no end to the multitasking that can be done.

The Big O

I've saved the best for last. And I bet you thought the sleeping orgasm was as good as it could possibly get, right? Now we talk about the Pregnant Orgasm. Wouldn't you just know that it would be different from a non-pregnant one? Orgasm is such a hard thing to describe and quantify, but I'll endeavor to do my best for my Girlfriends. After hundreds of hours of discussion with my Girlfriends on this subject (one of our favorites), we have consensus on three major points: First, if you are at all interested in sex, you can now get aroused much more quickly than ever before. Second, even though you are easily aroused, it will probably take you longer than before to achieve an orgasm. And third, you should take all the extra time you need because the pregnant orgasm is even more profound, longer-lasting, and accompanied by more aftershocks than any you've ever experienced before. While the initial impact is now measurable on the

Richter scale, you will have more that are strong enough to be considered measurable earthquakes themselves. Sometimes these aftershocks can be a little scary because they cause your uterus to seriously contract. Talk to your doctor about it, but most doctors are a little envious of your condition, and they'll probably agree that your pregnancy can take this kind of tossing and turning, and more.

10

Looking the Best You Can

Fashion

In the first edition of this book, I wrote something to the effect that the road to fashion hell began at the door of a maternity clothing store. I didn't hear much disagreement from readers, but the maternity fashion (previously an oxymoron) industry was mightily offended. One of the biggies refused to carry any of my books in its stores for a decade. Well, several visits to maternity stores during the last year of my research for this updated *Girlfriends' Guide,* particularly those sharing a building in midtown Manhattan across from the Four Seasons Hotel, have led me to reconsider my statement. I'm not exactly offering an olive branch, but I am willing to acknowledge what a difference a decade makes.

Water Shouldn't Roll Off Your Clothes

First of all, the fabrics have been vastly improved, at least in the more pricey stores. You used to be able to run through a maternity store with a torch and never start a fire because all the fabrics just melted into plastic puddles. Everything from faux-denim jeans to faux-linen suits had a shininess that just screamed polyester. Not anymore, my Girlfriends. Cotton, that wonderful, soft, absorbent, and breathable material, is all over the place now. Even organic cottons (meaning they weren't treated with pesticides or other chemicals during growth and processing) can be found in some chain stores and boutiques. Silks and linens abound, too, although most Girlfriends agree that these wrinkle beyond recognition and are best worn in air-conditioning. Best of all is the introduction of fabric blends that combine the comfort and drape of naturals with the fit, wrinkle resistance, and cleaning ease of synthetics . . . and no shine in sight, unless expressly intended! So if chiffons or gauzes or wool plaids are in fashion for the nonpreggers of the world, they can be in fashion for you, too.

"Dolce and Gabbana, Fendi, and Then Donna Karan, They Be Sharin' . . ."

Second, nonmaternity fashion designers and manufacturers now cater to the stylish mommies-to-be. Everybody from Diane von Furstenberg to St. John to Versace has outfitted an expectant celebrity. Remember Angelina in those gray and black suits when she attended summits at the United Nations? How about Catherine Zeta-Jones in all that black silk, boobies riding high and proud, accepting her Academy Award for *Chicago* while practically in labor? Gwen Stefani, who is already a fashion designer, came up with some of her best designs to clothe herself at the Grammys and the zillions of other photo ops, intentional or not, that besiege stars these days. There were Jennifer Garner and Gwyneth Paltrow and Heidi Klum simultaneously gestating and walking the red carpets and streets of LA and New York. Any *garmento* with half a brain for marketing had to realize that these fashionistas would need to be outfitted during their reproductions as well as during their film or record productions, and that their tastes were just as discriminating. Besides, as anyone who's ever seen signage on city buses knows, big things that move around town provide good opportunities to advertise. So if Britney found a cute T-shirt at Kitsons, the rest of us would notice within a couple of days and just have to have it.

The Elephant in the Room

The third big change in maternity fashion, and to me the most revolutionary of all, is the celebration of the bump. Ten years ago, the thought of wearing a little white tee that hugs the bust and belly and stops just below the navel with the printed message *Knocked Up* was sure to elicit remarks like "That's just gross" or "No one needs to see all that." Until the last few years, maternity clothes were designed to hide and camouflage the baby factory, rather like a termite tent keeping the whole messy structure under wraps. "Don't mind me," we seemed to be saying, "I'll just get this over with as quickly as possible and with minimal fuss or muss." Now fashion seems to be agreeing with the Girlfriends that this attitude is a recipe for personality disintegration, or at least for getting really, really resentful.

Recently, while getting my hair blown out, I was eye level with the belly of my pregnant stylist, Zoe. I could clearly see her tattoo, which used to sit right above her bikini but was now stretched out like the writing on a party balloon. I could also see the hole in her belly button where she'd removed her piercing because the gold ring wouldn't stay in as her button started reversing from an innie to an outie. She had on a muscle tee and some cotton gauchos with a rollover top that rolled under her tanned and tattied belly. She looked positively adorable and so hip. She seemed to be perfectly appropriate and "up-front" about what was going on with her, and it freed me to ask when she was due, which I'm usually too frightened to do in case I've guessed wrong. There it was for all to see—a baby that Zoe didn't expect but welcomed, as did her boyfriend. No stories about being "almost engaged" and not telling anyone until their parents knew. It was a fait accompli and it was nearly poking me in the eye. I so admired its candor.

Speaking of candor, my Girlfriend Cammie recently found an amazing dress online to wear to an LBDP (Little-Black-Dress Party). It was shirred in a thin, gauzy, black material that hugged her body down to her knees. Of course, being five feet nine helped her pull this off; I would have looked as wide as I was tall in the same dress. It showed off her bump, boobs, and booty and accentuated the curve in her back and under her belly, too. Now, that's a bold statement from any angle and sure to shock her parents and in-laws, but she was spectacular. This body consciousness is the natural extension of Girlfriends who grew up with Juicy sweats or Hardtails, and it's irresistible for its lack of fussiness. Fussiness used to be synonymous with pregnancy, and it's nice to see it go.

I've even noticed stylish girls intentionally violating the First Pregnancy Fashion Rule of Accessorizing by belting full dresses and tops *under* their belly. I remember trying that with my first pregnancy when I was in that in-between stage, where my maternity clothes were too big and my regular clothes were too small, and I was trying to control all the fabric in my black, collar-necked dress with a chic little raffia belt below my belly. My husband sat quietly on the bed watching me get more flustered, frantic, and sweaty, trying to find a look good enough to let me leave the house for a couple of hours without eliciting giggles and guffaws. Finally, he couldn't contain himself another moment and burst out laughing. "It looks like you've closed a volleyball up in your beach umbrella," he roared as he ran quickly to the bathroom. Coward. Little did I know my impetuous and desperate attempt to present myself as a still-fashionable woman would someday be vindicated, if only for a moment.

Fashionable and Fit (or Dressed like It)

One of the best things to happen to mommies-to-be was the yoga movement. Sure, yoga is a good form of fitness and relaxation for Girlfriends, whether they're pregnant or not, but more important are the soft, stretchy clothes that come along with its practice. (Don't hate the playah, you yoganistas. I've already confessed my reservations about exercise and pregnancy in chapter 8.) Christy Turlington came out with her clothing line during her yogic maternity years, and the forgiving stretch pants with rollover tops and slightly flared legs that fashionable yoginis adopted were addictive to the rest of us who were pregnant and still doing our sun salutes and downward dogs. Yoga girls in their prime often wear a cropped top or sports bra to complete their ensemble, and pregnant girls like Christy Turlington probably do, too. The more human among us wear the same outfit but put a long cotton tee or tunic over it—anything that doesn't fall over our heads to smother us while doing handstands (as if).

The look has made its way beyond yoga studios to chai tea latte pickups at Coffee Bean and Tea Leaf and then on to other errands. The clothes are so soft and stretchy and forgiving that, if most pregnant women had their way, they'd probably wear the same kind to work and dinner and the theater. Even now when I'm not pregnant, I crave sweats and other workout clothes that don't bind or wedge or chafe, and so do my Girlfriends.

What About Those of Us with Real Jobs?

As much as fashion has responded to the chic pregnant celebrities, it still has some work to do in the world of women who are in business, medicine, law, sales, and services, besides making babies. If we all lived at the beach, wore flip-flops or platform sandals, and could show up at work in clothes so sheer that our bras were considered part of the fashion statement, we'd be pretty well taken care of. But most of the cute stuff is overtly sexual, or long and sheer and romantic in a Malibu-by-way-of-the-Hamptons sort of way. And wonderful as jeans by 7 for All Mankind and

Paige Premium are, when hitched under the belly or with a panel over the belly, unless it's Casual Friday in Dogpatch, jeans are not generally considered the most direct way to break through the glass ceiling.

As a criminal attorney, my Girlfriend Rebecca is always meticulous in her dress. She says that her job is to look professional and pulled together without creating any distractions from the case at hand with loud prints or colors or too much skin. Try pulling *that* look off pregnant. While representing a client in court, Becca liked fitted jackets with skirts or trousers, with a flat, ballerina-type shoe or modest pump or boot. She is also apt to sweat profusely during her second and third trimesters as her Crock-Pot of a belly makes her hotter and hotter, so she needs fabrics that can breathe and absorb some of the dampness.

At first, she made do with her old styles in larger sizes, but by the time she got the jacket back from the tailor who'd shortened the sleeves of the size 10 she'd just bought, her back and boobs had put on another layer of "fuel" and she looked like the Incredible Hulk as she stretched the armhole. Or the bigger pants could fasten around her belly only if she pulled them up over the bump, thereby creating a wedgie that was unbearable, not to mention unattractive, or else pulled them below it and risked losing them if she let go of her tummy contraction for a moment. That's when she turned to maternity fashions and called me, crying, on her cell to ask for some direction.

Obviously, she didn't want to buy a whole new wardrobe that she'd wear for no more than six months, but she didn't also want to show up in the same outfit every single day. What was a Girlfriend to do? Separates! That's what we do. We build a core group comprising a dress, a skirt, pants, two or three tops, and a couple of jackets or wraps in complementary colors and call it a day.

There used to be a kit, much like those bed-in-a-bag sets of linens, that included a tunic, a tee, a skirt, and some pants, all made out of a knit fabric, and the whole shebang was either black, brown, or gray, as I recall. Macy's used to sell them, but I haven't seen them in years. Babystyle has taken the same idea and identified the five or six pieces of clothing that every mommy-to-be should have, such as a jean, a wrap dress, a tunic, and a pretty top and pants, and has shown variations on that theme to fit each woman's taste and wardrobe specifics. Best of all, these basics are not all the same drab color as the Belly Basics used to be.

Keep in mind that all of these pieces are maternity, not just bigger sizes of regular fashions. So even if tunics are fashionable for everybody this season, don't expect even the loosest nonmaternity ones to fit you for long. You're better off with one made of T-shirt cotton that drapes fetchingly and has room in front for your growing belly and boobs, as well as your booty, which will be wanting some cover of its own. Same with the wrap dresses. Ubiquitous as they are these days, do buy those made expressly for pregnancy. This will spare you the fashion don'ts of too much cleavage and a hem that rides up in front. In maternity fashion the rule is "There's a place for everything and everything in its place," and that applies to all body parts.

Pregnancy Fashion Challenges

Air, We Need Air

It takes a lot of calorie-burning to manufacture a baby or two in one's belly, and all that burning leads to a noticeable rise in a pregnant gal's core body temperature. On an episode of *Grey's Anatomy* a pregnant doctor says that unborn boys burn 10 percent more calories than girls do, so moms of little boys can really feel steam heat. (And, yes, I do get a lot of my information from television, but only from the professionals.) Add that to the unpredictable fluctuations of temperature caused by the ebbs and flows of hormones through your body, and you have the recipe for a private greenhouse effect. Not only do you have the predictable sweat under the arms, but for those of us who were formerly flat-chested, there is the wondrous and weird experience of feeling rivulets dripping down between our big new breasts. Some of us even find moisture collecting *under* our bustline when we lift them up to scratch or marvel in their weight. And even if most girls don't like to talk about such indignities, if taking a lie detector test, we'd all have to confess to the occasional sweat between our chafing thighs.

Another consideration, just between us girls, is a pregnant woman's increased vaginal, and occasionally breast, secretions. As my Girlfriend Greta remarked recently, "Nobody tells you how damp and swollen everything gets. And I mean *everything*!" Well, we're telling you now. Just writing this has me reaching for a paper fan and cotton panties! Now you can see why natural, absorbent fabrics that breathe are so welcome in today's maternity fashions. Even in the dead of winter, you will want to feel a bit of a breeze whenever possible.

Start with the garments closest to your skin: panties, bras, and undershirts. These are where you want cotton and plenty of it. Even if you're still wearing your thongs, make sure that at least the lining is cotton, or wear a breathable minipad. It's great to be able to wear sexy maternity jeans by all the hip designers, but you may find that all that stands between you and Mycolog cream is cotton. By the way, yeast infections are particularly common during pregnancy, and you should never use any over-the-counter treatments without talking to your obstetrician—but I digress.

Cat-Scratch Fever

Another phenomenon of pregnancy is the urge to scratch your belly and boobs. I don't know where the urge comes from, but my Girlfriends and I all reported the sublime feeling at the end of the day of taking off all binding clothes and having a good stretch and scratch. I, the descendant of Irish and Norwegian people who were melanin-challenged, would look as if I'd made love to the Wolverine by the time I was finished. The urge was irresistible, no matter what fabrics I'd worn, but I did notice that the itching was exacerbated by synthetic fibers that bound me under my breasts or across my belly in the form of elastic. I recommend that, in addition to getting new, professionally fitted bras during pregnancy, Girlfriends get their foundations in cotton, or at least cotton blends. Hey, you're buying new bras every couple of months anyway (or should be), you might as well sacrifice some of the itchy lacy bits for the next few months.

The cotton wife-beater, or whatever you call thin, sleeveless T-shirts in your neck of the woods, is heaven's most recent fashion gift to mommies-to-be. Everybody, pregnant or not, layers her tops these days, and the plain, white tee is the universal primary layer. You may have to look for slightly roomier and longer versions of the old standby, but it will still be your fashion friend. With the cotton tee close to your skin, any second layer will be fine. Go ahead and get the taffeta ruffles, the satin blends, or the rayons that look so cute and spunky, and feel safe and comfortable in the second skin that cotton provides.

If the Baby Is in My Belly, Why Is My Booty So Big?

After four trips up and down the maternity mountain, I've realized that my fantasy of being pregnant took me only into the second trimester. I was so impatient during the first trimester to have a real bump, one that looked undeniably pregnant rather than like bloat or too many biscuits with my gravy; but I never realized that the bump was often accompanied by the butt, the boobs, the arms, the face, and the legs. If my belly were the only thing to grow, I could have embraced my low-rise jeans and got a couple of longer shirts and called it a day.

But for me, pregnancy was a full-body experience—I was pregnant from my glowing face to my disappearing ankles. There wasn't much to do about the face except rely on Girlfriends to keep me from cutting my hair into a *Rosemary's Baby* pixie in a moment of hormone-induced hysteria. My upper arms, however, were a crisis unto themselves. I recently looked at pictures taken at a couple of my baby showers, and here's what I learned: Sleeveless and nine months pregnant is not my best look. Pressing those hams against my sides made them look bigger than my thighs. And for Girlfriends like Kristi, who got mysterious tiny, red bumps on her upper arms, this was adding insult to injury. Clearly, sleeves that come down to just above the elbow can be our friend.

The interview with Britney Spears and Matt Lauer will go down in infamy, if not as a cautionary tale about chewing gum on network television, then as an example of how pregnancy can beef up a girl's chest and shoulders so much that she looks like a linebacker. I experienced this myself, so this is no disrespect for Brit. It's just worth noting because spaghetti straps and tight armholes may only make the problem appear worse. Fashion is our friend when we embrace its ability to fool the eye. Breaking up the broad expanse from cleavage to clavicle with a neckline that extends straight across from armpit to armpit can be far more tidy-looking than the low V-neck of many casual tops. You don't need to button up to there to look pulled together, but only the Girlfriends with the smallest of breasts can get by with minimal bust support and full disclosure of the cleavage. If there's a noticeable cleavage line that's longer than four inches from the top of the crease to the top of the blouse, you risk letting the milk factory, not your belly or your beaming face, become the featured attraction, especially when sitting in a chair and leaning slightly forward toward your interviewer.

Another sign that it's time to adjust your fashion silhouette is when your bust starts to rest on your belly like a walrus on a rock. The optical effect of that merger is like that of the prow of a ship, and the fashion antidote is an empire waist or a band of some kind breaking up that line. Gwen Stefani wore the most beautiful dresses when she was pregnant: The fabrics were brilliantly exotic and finely detailed. But if you look closely, all those dresses had a visual contrast in cut and color between her bust and her baby belly, not to mention a bit of a sleeve toward the end. She never looked massive and shapeless, but rather chic, sexily voluptuous, and irresistibly pregnant with a bump that looked reassuringly proportionate. You might choose an empire cut or make one yourself with a belt or ribbon or tied shrug. However you break up the visual line between bump and boobs, just know that doing so can go miles toward distinguishing you from Quasimodo. Keep this in mind, you Girlfriends expecting multiples, because this fashion tidbit will stand you in particularly good stead as your girth expands.

People love a baby bump. You'll want to protect it, rub it, and rest your arms on it. Your mate may be inclined to massage it and put an ear to it to see if anything can be heard. Your best Girlfriend will probably be willing to place a hand on the spot where you last felt a kick and let it rest lightly there in hopes of feeling the next one. A pregnant belly is one of the most irresistible sights in nature. For this reason, it's also a particularly complex fashion consideration. Way back in the "olden days" of my first pregnancy, a woman put several protective layers between her baby and the outside world. If someone had suggested that I wear jeans that buttoned under my belly and a blouse that flowed loosely to just below my navel, I would have felt faint. The thought of a breeze blowing my top up to reveal any of my pregnancy, or of some stranger being able to slip a hand up underneath it to touch the tight skin of my belly, would have been so anxiety-provoking that I would have taken to my bed. In those dark ages, my Girlfriends and I wore pants and skirts with belly panels that came well up and over our bumps or dresses that draped from the collar to the hem, with an empire style thrown in now and then.

These days, the belly is often out there for all to see (and some to touch), especially among the Girlfriends who appear in *Us* or *People*. One thing that the hip bumps have in common seems to be a tan. Whether it be UV-induced or painted on, the smooth brown belly is fashionable. Call me crazy, but I think pregnant women are most apt to allow their tummy to be out in the elements when it's tan, rather than a virgin to sun and cosmetics. I guess a little airbrush tan never hurt any belly, but the risks of sunbathing still apply to pregnant women—even if they are suffering from hormone hysteria—and the Girlfriends give it a thumbs-down.

No matter how you feel about the brazen belly, almost all pregnant Girlfriends hesitate a moment when their belly buttons begin to claim a life of their own. Like a Butterball-turkey timer, my navel popped, changing from innie to outie by my third trimester. Let me hasten to add that it always went back to innie after the baby was born—so you won't always look like a giant nipple. But the more it protruded, the more squeamish I became. Not only was I repelled by the thought of a complete stranger, or even a casual acquaintance, running a hand over it, I myself was unwilling to touch it, except with a washcloth in the shower. My Girlfriend Mary used to put a big Band-Aid over her button every morning and it worked pretty well, but pulling it off every night was irritating to her skin. I recently found the most ingenious solution online, called Popper Stoppers, and I'm truly impressed by American ingenuity. These superthin, latex-free second skins claim to adhere to the skin but not the navel, and to be invisible under clingy satins or smooth tees. By the seventh or eighth month, however, almost all moms with a sense of style (or a modicum of modesty) have turned to tunics, long shirts, or maternity tops, grateful for the added coverage and adjusted proportions of clothes designed to accommodate a baby belly.

Particularly fabulous is the camouflaging of the hips and fanny that these tops provide. One undeniable risk of clingy tops or dresses is not just their tendency to accentuate the odd shapes of a pregnant belly in its final days, but also that they are just as attracted to a Girlfriend's bottom. Once again, let me sing the praises of a three-way mirror, Girlfriends. Never forget that the backside may be growing nearly as quickly as the front. Maybe it's part of the milk factory's need to store fuel, or maybe it's nature's way of buttressing our struts to make sure we can support the new addition, but it's there. I remember an anthropology class in college that showed pictures of gorilla moms walking on feet and knuckles with their babies riding atop their haunches. We may not drag our knuckles anymore, but the haunches seem to be our evolutionary holdovers, and I used them as perches for my older kids in subsequent pregnancies.

As I've mentioned before, a pregnant woman retains an awful lot of water, and after a long day you may notice that gravity brings most of it to your feet and legs. My Girlfriend Andrea, who was pregnant with her son during the dog days of summer, described her feet as meat loaves and her toes as Vienna sausages. My Girlfriend Caroline recently told me that she had "cankles" in the last days of gestating her twins—her calves and ankles had mushed into one undifferentiated appendage. This is when your Girlfriends who've already limped a mile in these moccasins have two things to tell you: First, put your feet up whenever you can. Second, think motorcycle boots, long hemlines, and dark stockings. Flip-flops or Birkenstocks may feel great in private, but they have nothing to offer to the stylish mom.

Live for Today

You will find more than enough fashionable clothing to get you through your nine (ten) months of pregnancy and several weeks postpartum. You will also notice that the best clothes cost as much as their nonmaternity counterparts. A pair of $200 jeans that you can justify with the knowledge that you'll get a couple of years' enjoyment out of them is one thing; their maternity-cut counterparts for the same price are a lot harder to wrap your credit card around. Think about it: You may not even need new jeans (especially if you do the old trick of expanding your regular jeans' waistline by wrapping a hair elastic around the button, through the buttonhole, and back around the button) until you're about five months pregnant.

Spending a couple hundred for maternity jeans that you'll wear for four or five months can give you pause. One thing the Girlfriends can tell you unequivocally is this: Never justify spending a lot of money on a maternity outfit by saying, "This is so cute that I can even wear it after the baby is born." If you wear any maternity clothes four weeks after your baby is born, I offer to eat them, Girlfriend! There is no pleasure more profound than putting all those outfits into a box and giving them the old heave-ho after your belly disappears, even if you're still big everywhere else.

Pass It On

My Girlfriends and I developed a maternity lending library of fashion. Most women have more than one child, which means that the cost of buying a few key maternity clothes can be amortized against two or three seasons of wear. If you find two or three reproductive Girlfriends, whether at your obstetrician's, your prepared-childbirth classes, or in your neighborhood, you can form a clothing "co-op." I did it with three Girlfriends and we ended up getting a fifth member of the co-op when a surprise pregnancy made her one of us.

No matter when you conceive, you are bound to need one dress for a holiday/event. This can be expensive when purchased as a one-off. But if you agree to buy an LBD (Little Black Dress) and your Girlfriend Amy buys the festive, sexy party dress, and your Girlfriend Mindy buys a long sweater wrap, and your Girlfriend Corki buys two pairs of roll-top trousers, you're more than halfway to a fabulous maternity wardrobe.

My Girlfriends of the same reproductive eras as I realized what a treasure trove we had when we combined our resources, but not until several of us had gone through our first pregnancies as solo acts and had sunk a lot of money into outfits that were only briefly, or never, worn and then put in storage. Predictably, other Girlfriends got pregnant with their firsts, and we returned for our second, third, and fourth trips down Maternity Lane and pulled those clothes out of storage. Soon we realized that with a bit of planning, even two Girlfriends who were due virtually the same day could share a wardrobe. So many maternity clothes are cut so roomy and forgiving and adjustable that Girlfriends who are size 4, 6, or even 10 when not pregnant can share the same clothes while pregnant. The biggest variation we noticed was in hemlines and cuffs, so we all bought our own double-stick tape to temporarily "alter" the lending library's clothes.

The total loss of short-term memory that is a hallmark of new mommyhood made the reappearance of the same outfits that we'd passed on only a year ago surprising and thrilling. Even after my own four were born and my gestation buddies were hanging up their maternity saddles, we had younger Girlfriends who inherited our communal wardrobe for several more babies. Eventually the collection included nursing bras, belly bands, surplus newborn diapers, and boppy pillows and bassinets. A little laundering and antiseptic soap rendered these things perfectly useful and economical. It was brilliant.

We Deserve to Swim

The single most comfortable place for a seriously pregnant woman to be is in water. I was addicted to my bathtub when I was pregnant (up until my water broke or I passed my mucus plug, of course). Being buoyant was such a relief, and the comfort of refreshing water that wasn't too hot or too cold was so soothing that I could understand some women's desire for a water birth (though I couldn't see myself doing it). And since normal pregnancies last forty weeks, chances are we'll all be blossoming at some time that calls for a bathing suit.

I don't think I passed through this fashion wicket successfully once in my forty months of gestation. I am one of those girls who gain one pound and show it in their thighs. I yearned to be obviously pregnant and lightly tanned and frolicking along the shore in a bikini, like Elle MacPherson or Victoria "Posh Spice" Beckham. Instead, being of fair and freckled skin and showing enough cellulite to suggest I'd been pelted on my backside with cottage cheese, I tried to stay as far from all water recreation as possible. When I absolutely had to, I wore regular one-piece bathing suits in the beginning with a pareo always attached to my tushy, but eventually my boobs needed the support of built-in bras (and I mean BIG ones), and my belly pulled the suit so far forward that the leg holes looked revoltingly revealing.

By my third pregnancy, with my second son, I met up with my in-laws to take all the kids to Disney World . . . in JULY! Orlando in the summer at seven months pregnant was a hardship only a woman who has walked in those moccasins, with two tiny children in tow, can know. I never cooled off—not in the room, not at night, not in Epcot, nowhere. The pools and pretend beaches surrounding our hotel were calling to me like the Nestea plunge and I wanted to respond, so I bought a navy-blue-and-white maternity one-piece. Nautical and maternal are linked in some way I've never figured out; maybe the thinking is "If it looks like a ship, treat it like a ship." It may or may not have had a panel or skirtish thing, I don't recall, because I experienced post-traumatic stress syndrome over it and have no memory of the entire time. I have since seen pictures, however, and I've learned that, first, we women are entitled to swim no matter how imperfect we feel, and second, by the sixth or seventh gestational month, unless you are a supermodel over six feet tall or a celebrity with an eating disorder, most of us Girlfriends just won't be rapturously showing off any bathing suit.

The good news is, by that time in your pregnancy no one is really looking at you and saying, "Look how pudgy and lumpy she is." They are saying, "Isn't she just adorable, that little mommy? She looks so healthy." We are no longer held to Nicole Ritchie or Lindsay Lohan standards because it's obvious we're busy doing something else far more important, thank you very much. I mean it, Girlfriend; nobody cares except you (and maybe a shell-shocked partner, who hasn't said one thing right for months now anyway). Go ahead and smear your oils and anti-stretch-mark potions on and massage your belly right out in public if you want; I guarantee they all secretly wish they could be you (or your close personal friend).

Ten years after I wrote the first edition of this book, I can enthusiastically say that you have more choices of maternity bathing suits now. They have lost the tenting and skirts of the previous decade, and sleekly support your belly with invisible panels. They also architecturally defy gravity by holding your heavy bosom up and off that belly, which actually makes you look smaller because the total mass is broken up, thus making each part look smaller. Not to mention that it's nice to take a load off your back for a while.

Tankinis, one of the best new styles made for the preggers, are cut longer than the nonmaternity versions to cover up most of the belly, while offering more booty coverage and lifting that up off your thighs, too. Those attributes are so good that you may want to wear a bathing suit even in the comfort of your own house. (More about undergarments that achieve those things later in this chapter.) Oh, yeah, in hindsight, my advice is to skip the navy-and-white entirely, unless you're a merchant marine or in the navy. Now is the time for color.

You should boldly encourage admiring looks from strangers because you are Superwoman! You are growing an entire person inside of you all by yourself! You are to be applauded whenever people see you, for you are following your biological imperative and moving the DNA into the future. Plus, vivid colors and prints can distract from the cottage-cheese effect.

One last thing about bathing suits and maternity: You can burn in places you never knew you had, not to mention that the skin reacts completely differently to the sun and other elements when pregnant. So use a sunscreen every day and a sunblock on the sensitive areas: bosom, upper legs around bottom of the bathing suit, and, need I even say it, face. Chloasma, or the "mask of pregnancy," which many mommies get while gestating, is made garish with the darkening effect of the sun. Sunbathing is so unnecessary these days anyway, with richer and deeper tans from lotions and airbrushing. And take it from this mommy veteran, you never want to be asked if you're the child's mother or grandmother, so treat your complexion now the way you'll treat your baby's bottom . . . when you get your hands on it.

The Garments Under the Garments: "I See London, I See France, I See Someone's Underpants!"

I know they are still sold in stores, but I haven't found a single woman who wears big, over-the-belly maternity panties in nearly twenty years of prying into private matters. Thongs are popular with many of my pregnant Girlfriends, but I can't bear them even when I'm not pregnant. Far more comfortable to many of the fashionable pregnant set are the thin, lace elastic hipsters or bikinis such as those delicious hues of Hanky Panky or Cosabella. Pricey they may be, but you can get less expensive versions that are equally wonderful at Victoria's Secret. All you're really looking for is something with a cotton liner and a smoothing band of elastic to grip that uncharted territory between your belly and your pubic bone. And lovely bright colors can be a mood elevator of the nonprescription kind.

Speaking just among us Girlfriends, even if you, like I, often prefer going "commando," it's not usually a good hygiene choice during maternity. I believe I've mentioned before that things get rather, how should I say it, *tropical* down there. Between the intimacy your thighs must be experiencing just now, the added fluids of perspiration, and vaginal secretions (there's just no dainty way of saying this), you could probably bake bread down there. "But that's exactly why being panty-free is so irresistible," you may say. And to that I say, knock yourself out if you're wearing cotton, breathable drawstring pants or you're naked except for a tampon (which is *not* recommended by the Girlfriends) or if you're sitting on a beach towel somewhere. Any other scenario might just not be as *fresh* as a Girlfriend would like.

Girdles, Slings, and Panty Hose, Oh My

You might think that girdles and panty hose would be the last thing a nice, big pregnant woman would want to wear, unless of course you are as white, freckled, and blue-veined as I. They sound stiflingly hot, restrictive, unattractive (the supreme buzz kill), and maybe even not good for the baby. To my Girlfriend Andrea, the worst thing about having anything over her belly was her inability to get in a good tummy scratch from time to time. And yet many of my most rational and free-spirited Girlfriends have made a good case for slipping into the shield and support of panty hose and girdles or body smoothers.

First, as my Girlfriend Sheree told me, until we're about five months pregnant, most of us don't look unmistakably preggie. We could just as easily have put on the undifferentiated (read: lumpy) weight gain by being premenstrual and chugging a few too many venti Frappuccinos. By the sixth month, the pregnancy is big enough to provide the horizontal tent pole that gives us that unmistakable shape of gestators. But until then, slimmers and control tops can give a smoother line to our silhouettes, especially, Sheree explains, in the booty and upper-thigh area.

Though I might sound like a wimp when I say this, this is definitely something you should talk to your OB about, Girlfriend. I don't know much about our bodies and their fluids, but common sense would make me ask, "What happens if the elastic waistbands or the tight legs that most of these slimmers have get too tight?" Can they cut off blood flow? Do they keep the retained water, well, *retained*? Does that mean that when you take them off in the evening, your arms and legs are puffed up like water balloons and your fingers like pork links? To paraphrase Kelly Ripa, I'm just saying . . .

In the last couple of months of pregnancy, or even sooner with multiples (twins or more), so many Girlfriends complain about back pain. Just think about the stereotypical pregnant woman: She stands with her shoulders back and drooped, her big belly pulling her lower spine forward, and leaning back on her heels to keep from falling on her face. Gosh, I felt that way with my third and fourth babies, and they were barely seven pounds and came one at a time.

And it's not just the posture that is being challenged. All that pressure on the nerves going under the belly and into the hips gives millions of Girlfriends sciatica, which sends alternating firelike pain and total numbness down one or both legs. This condition usually goes away upon delivery or shortly thereafter, but it's the devil when you have it.

My Girlfriend Peggy had sciatica with all three of her babies, and it got a little worse with each subsequent pregnancy because her abdominal muscles weren't as taut as before and her pelvic floor might have been a little traumatized by then.

Peggy wept a lot toward the end of her first pregnancy, but by her second and third she used a belly sling to redistribute some of the belly weight to her back and shoulders. I've checked several online sites that sell such contraptions, including everything from custom-sized girdles to belly holders that have straps that go up and over the shoulders or criss-cross against the back. All the customer endorsements enthusiastically declared that the women couldn't have survived their last trimester, their triplets, or their baby's dropping into birth position without these devices.

These same customers also couldn't say enough about how these things relieved a problem I hadn't even thought could be helped: incontinence! My Girlfriends and I are unanimous in our dumb acceptance that a very pregnant mommy's bladder might as well wear a *Kick Me* sign, for all the abuse it takes from Little Junior. You know the feeling; you have to pee so badly that you're in tears, yet when you sit to relieve yourself, there's just a piddle or two. We have just accepted it like turkeys who don't know enough to come in out of the rain, but instead look up at the sky for some sort of explanation, only to drown as the rain fills their open beaks. The manufacturers of these products say that we need not drown in our own piddle ever again, and if your doctor agrees, you may find it to be true. I would have thought that Mother Nature would have provided us with strong enough girdles of our own in our belly and back musculature, but maybe she wasn't considering so many twins, triplets, and quads, nor for so many of us to have our first baby in our thirties and even forties. Maybe you have to respond to technology with more technology. Just promise me you'll ask your doctor.

For Those Big Titties

Breasts, glorious breasts. I like to think of them as prizes for the "other babies" in our lives. You know how when a smart Girlfriend goes to visit her Girlfriend's second or subsequent baby, she always brings a gift for the siblings to make them feel included and loved? Well, I think the arrival of the Titty Fairy is not just to prepare the milk factory for its new client, but to amuse the father, to make him feel included and loved. Truly, they are the gifts that keep on giving, and giving and giving . . . often until you feel that they're taking over your life.

They're extremely heavy, often between two and five pounds! And like huge juicy apples, they follow Newton's law of gravity and tend to drop. Your mission, should you choose to accept it, is to defy gravity with the proper support of a bra, thus keeping the *National Geographic* knee-length boobies at bay. I don't want to hear how you've never worn a bra with more than a single hook in the back or an underwire, Girlfriend. Get over yourself! You will need a bra to lift your growing breasts up and off your belly (where, I PROMISE you, they will eventually come to rest) and to protect the fragile musculature that is trying to hold the twins up near your chest. You will also need to change your bra size an average of three times in the nine (ten) months of pregnancy.

So don't go telling me that you're still wearing your regular bras, just on a wider hook, Girlfriend. You're not just wider around in general; your cup size is changing. If you stick to your old bras and just let them out through all the rows of hooks or, worse, get bra extenders, pretty soon your boobies will be spilling out over the top of the lacy cups and your shoulders will have permanent grooves where the skinny straps go.

Oprah has had several shows on how essential it is for any woman with breasts big enough to fill a champagne glass to get a bra professionally fitted IN PERSON by an experienced fitter, and to use that fitter's help in selecting the right underpinnings for you.

Never in your life will that be more important than now. This is when a wider back strap with fasteners three to four down and three across can make the difference between you and a humpback or chronic neck pain. A broader band underneath your bosom can prevent that suffocating feeling that your lungs are being crushed by the tourniquet of your old bra's skinny band. This is when the old Playtex phrase *to lift and separate* might have relevance to your life.

Pushed together like a giant loaf of bread, your breasts can make a shelf that seems to descend from your shoulders, looking like a gigantic growth below your neck, Girlfriend! Separating your twins into individuals and supporting them with proper underwire, and whatever other trussing is available, can restore them to their rightful position as objects of envy and desire. And if that's not exactly your goal, then you'll at least be happy with the comfort and relief you'll feel.

Yes, maternity bras are widely available, but most of those convert to nursing bras when the time comes. Because of the accommodations for exposing the nipples and then covering them back up, often with an absorbent pad tucked in, I preferred to save the mommy bras for after the baby was born. Plenty of nonpregnant women with large breasts are buying bras by the minute, and you can piggyback on their demands for style, sex appeal, and affordability right up to the time you need to bare your breast for a truffle-sniffer like your newborn. The most important things are:

1. Try the bra on with an experienced fitter, or barring that, with a Girlfriend who has kids and knows that it has a function other than enticement.

2. Allow for change in cup size and circumference of chest. Remember, your entire torso is getting upholstered with a protective layer of fat and water, not just your breasts, and so all sizes will need to be reconsidered.

3. Make sure that the bust is held up by more than your bra's shoulder straps. A well-constructed bra will split some of the weight to the back with a wider band. You can tell if this band is doing its job by trying on the bra and pulling the back of the strap down to the same latitude as the front part. If it rides up high in back, it's not pulling its load AND it doesn't fit right.

4. You deserve black lace and you should get it. Even nursing bras come in sweet colors and sexy ones, too. If you can't find them at your local mall, go on-line to one of the major department stores or lingerie retailers. Just make sure that you have some idea of your new size before stocking up on several you haven't tried on. Go back to the mall and try on any ugly old thing and get a fit, then you'll be better able to order online for the cute, hot stuff.

5. Don't get attached to your bras. Even if you have judiciously bought bras that had some growth in them, few of us are really prepared for the size, shape, and weight (not to mention the temperature; but maybe that was just me) of third-trimester and postdelivery breasts. You can't predict this kind of mutiny, so you must be light on your feet and aware of when your old bras no longer have the twins in control. You will have to buy bras again, this late in pregnancy. The good news is, unlike with maternity clothes, you *will* wear your big bras beyond pregnancy, especially if they are nursing bras.

6. Save them. Long after you've stopped nursing and your breasts look, at least to you, smaller and less spunky than before you got pregnant, it will be hard to imagine them ever again knowing their former pregnancy glory. You'd be right, of course—UNTIL you get pregnant again, at which time you will become just as perky and undeniably present as before. You'll want those big old bras back in your drawers then, big-time.

The Fashion We Never Take Off

It's All About the Hair

My hair matters. I mean REALLY matters, in a sick, narcissistic way that I'm ashamed to admit. If my hair is clean, professionally blown dry, and bouncy to the point of eliciting compliments from strangers, it's a good day. Even if I get fired from my job, my husband leaves me, and my car is stolen, it's a good day. As long as I look good in the unemployment line, divorce court, or at the police station, I can take the other insignificant difficulties in my blown-and-bouncy stride. On the other hand, if my hair is flat, the color is oxidized, and I've gone one too many days without shampooing, you could tell me I've won the lottery and just need to drive to the corner market to pick up the money, and I wouldn't go.

In that regard, it's almost all good news. Sure, you might find you have to wash it more when you're pregnant, but that's a small price to pay for the thickness and health of your 'do. First, your body is in high gear, with its juices flowing and blood churning through the baby maker. That in itself would probably contribute to the good condition and growth of your hair, but another small miracle occurs during pregnancy: You stop shedding hair (or at least you shed much less of it), so usually there's a lot more to work with.

"I Could Just Dye!"

All this accelerated growth leads to one of the first big motherhood decisions you'll make: Should you continue to color your hair when you're pregnant? One school of thought that many moms-to-be subscribe to says that artificial dyes of any sort could be transmitted through the hair follicles and pores of the scalp and get into the placental blood and make your baby a bottle blond—no, just kidding—could make your baby slightly polluted in some way. OK, that's about all I have to say about that school of thought because that's about all I've ever found out about it. I never wanted to have so much information that it would get in the way of my decision making. My Girlfriend Garbo, an Italian beauty with big brown eyes and, yes, Garbo's platinum hair, announced early on that she would stay fabulously blond because it was only fair; after all, the baby was stealing her figure, her mind, and her ability to see her own feet.

I stayed naturally brunette with my first baby, but then again, I was still free of grays, and after three years of infertility, I would sacrifice anything to keep that baby. By the other babies, however, I got much more cavalier and vain. Not only did I keep up with my highlights, but I drank coffee, took Tylenol from time to time, and occasionally used artificial sweetener. So sue me—but get in line behind my kids' lawyers!

A couple of my Girlfriends compromised by eliminating any hair colors with peroxide and sticking to the darker pigments. Others stopped using permanent color for the nine (ten) months of pregnancy. Still others used products made from plants and berries and such. You can imagine how effective that was at eliminating any premature grays. . . . I support any choice a mommy makes for the baby in her belly. I did, however, notice that these Girlfriends unanimously ran for their bleaching, permanent, and vivid-colored hair dyes as soon as they could get to a salon. I'm just saying, if bark and tea are such good hair-coloring agents, why don't you see Louis Licari using them?

It's Nothing Permanent

Fashion is fickle, and as I write this book, perms are about as popular as stick-shift cars. Still, I've seen them come and go before and assume they will again, so this little bit on perms during pregnancy needs to be written. Besides, perms are also known as straighteners, and those are almost always in fashion somewhere—so this advice goes for them, too. PREGNANT HAIR WILL NOT "TAKE" A PERMANENT STRAIGHTENER OR CURLER EVENLY. In fact, it may not even take at all. Sorry, but this is just the way it is. I don't know why it happens, but you just have to trust the Girlfriends on this one. Get some clip-on extensions, wear a ponytail, and be ready to blow-dry for hours or to commit to hot rollers until you have given birth—and in some cases, quit breast-feeding—until you get your old head back. I don't even think you have to wait for the pregnant hairs to fall out or grow out—I think the old stuff just starts cooperating when the progesterone calms down.

All the Other Furry Places

It only makes sense that if the hair on your head is on overdrive, so is the hair under your arms, on your face, and, yes, *down there*. In fact, many of us grow peach fuzz on our jaws and cheeks. My Girlfriend Michele had fur high on her back, between her shoulders. Since Michele is a real blonde, this was only amusing to her. My brunette and olive-complected Girlfriend Soraya hated it when the same thing happened to her. I remember looking down at my bare breasts one morning and seeing a piece of lint or string on my chest. I nearly fainted when I tried to pick it off, only to discover that it was growing from my nipple!

Waxing is the logical solution, but you are certainly learning by now that nothing is that easy when you're pregnant. First of all, many experienced waxers say that yanking the hairs out by their roots is particularly painful when you have PMS or when you're pregnant. I don't know about you, but that was an extra pain I was willing to endure by about the third month. I live in Los Angeles, where I have Girlfriends from many ethnic groups, and another form of hair removal I've seen is called threading. Women who know this old technique work two threads around a hair and roll them to pull it out almost painlessly—I'm told. My Girlfriend Soraya ran to her threader as soon as her peach fuzz appeared on her cheeks and upper lip, and I never even knew that she'd grown a little furrier.

The bikini area's hair became of little interest to me once I could no longer see it. No matter what cute little design my waxer had created down there, I'm pretty sure it was unrecognizable with extra hair growth and all that stretching. My "landing strip" probably looked more like a baseball diamond by about my fifth month. Besides, I'd already noticed an unmistakable swelling in my labia, and a close-up view with a mirror revealed that my pinkies had turned a purplish blue. Right then, I decided I needed to grow as much hair down there as I could to camouflage them.

Skin—Our Body's Biggest Organ

In the first and last (and occasionally second) trimesters, you may find your coloring a little blotchy or even kind of green. The blotch is probably from the increased circulation, which can give your face a flush. The green is usually the result of not getting enough sleep and throwing up several times a day. This should pass after the first three months. In the meantime, keep concealer, those blotting papers, and mouthwash in your everyday bag.

The biggest skin issue experienced by the Girlfriends during pregnancy is *chloasma* or "the mask of pregnancy." It's a pigment irregularity that usually afflicts the forehead, cheeks, and nose. Think of it as being the Lone Ranger and getting a reverse tan; every place the mask touches is brown and all the other places aren't. This isn't unusual or bad in any way; it's just another hit to the vanity bone when it's already feeling bruised.

Sunlight only makes matters worse, so opt for sunblocks, not sunscreens. Look for the blocks with barriers such as zinc oxide (it's invisible now, so don't panic) to keep *all* sun off your face. You can apply all the tints and bronzes you want over it, but now's as good a time as ever to face up to the diminishing ozone layer and begin setting an example for your child that suntans are sun damage. Chloasma will clear up on its own after delivery, but not right away. You might want to consult a dermatologist about prescribing a bleaching cream or something to get rid of it faster, but make sure to ask first.

Just as pregnancy can make your pigment do weird things, it can also apply the same black magic to your moles and freckles. The freckles are just a few more things to bleach after delivery, but the moles should be watched carefully. We all know that a mole that suddenly changes in color, shape, or size needs to be checked out by a dermatologist. And because pregnancy seems to be an extrafertile season for moles, extra vigilance is recommended. I don't know about you, but I've been leaning toward getting those suckers removed whether they change or not, and I've been doing the same with my kids—but not until they are at least twelve years old, so calm yourself, Girlfriend.

One last mention about possible assaults on your skin when you're pregnant: Many of us, including me, get congested in pregnancy (consider yourself a giant mucous membrane while baby-making) and blow our noses so often that we get all chapped around our nostrils. First, wash your hands or Purell them before you touch your nose and after you blow. Second, use a simple moisturizer with sunblock to soothe and smoothe the area before applying more concealer. I made up the third thing myself, but it seems to help and couldn't hurt (ask your doctor anyway): I applied Polysporin ointment to the area at night after I washed my face. As my Girlfriend Stephanie discovered, pregnant women are just ripe for yeast— she got a mild infection in those indented spaces beside her nostrils. I'm not blaming anybody here, but I think a little more hand washing and protection of that area might have helped. . . . Not to worry, however, the doctor gave her a safe cream to clear it right up.

Things to Keep in Mind About Pregnancy Style

1. Many people, even in this enlightened age, find obvious evidence of reproduction slightly unnerving. With that in mind, keep cleavage, thighs, and bare bellies at least fifteen feet outside their personal space.

2. No matter how frantic you are to find a shirt that still fits today, don't fake it by wearing a bodysuit that snaps between your legs and stretches the legs up to your navel. (E.g., Katie Holmes, *Star,* April.)

3. Don't be a snob about where you find your clothes at this time. You'll only be wearing most of them for three or four months and then burning some of them in a postpartum moment.

4. Borrow anything you can. Better still, organize your reproductive Girlfriends into a maternity fashion cooperative. Catalog all the clothes, furniture, and accessories, and appoint a "librarian" to make sure that they're all returned after use, or else a penalty should be charged.

5. Really use the faux bump that maternity stores provide in most dressing rooms. Go ahead and strap that baby on and have a giggle with your Girlfriends about how you'd look pregnant if you were a supermodel.

6. Remember, even the maternity models who are actually pregnant in those pregnancy fashion layouts aren't usually booked after their fifth or early sixth month because they grow too fast and in too many places.

7. Find your look and stick to it. Now is not the time to experiment. If it's red lipstick and tunics, claim it and call it a day.

8. Don't leave home without spending at least ninety seconds in front of a three-way mirror. Your backside has a mind of its own, and you'll be the last to know its intentions until it's extremely embarrassing.

9. Spend the big bucks on your bras. They're carrying precious cargo while you carry the other precious cargo.

10. Buy one great LBD, preferably from a maternity store. Since average gestation is nine (ten) months, you are certain to be obviously pregnant for at least one major holiday or occasion. If you can't afford it, email all your mommy Girlfriends and their Girlfriends for a loan, because almost anything that's black, relatively little, and resembles a dress can probably fit you. Besides, they'll be thrilled to get that investment to pay off again.

11

Partners of Pregnant Women

A PREGNANT WOMAN is tremendously tempted to get so involved with her own emotions, thoughts, and worries that she has little time or interest in acknowledging how her partner is coping with the pregnancy. This is completely understandable, in my estimation; after all, we are the ones inhabited by an alien, we are the ones with hormones splashing around like Niagara Falls, and we are the ones who will have to somehow deliver the goods. All the partners have to deal with is *us*—but therein lies the problem. Dealing with us can be a demanding and frightening task, judging by what my Girlfriends' mates have told me. In fact, one of them suggested that I subtitle this chapter WHO ARE YOU AND WHAT HAVE YOU DONE WITH MY WOMAN?

Gone is the woman he fell for. Not only doesn't she look the same, she doesn't act anything like her old self. And to many a man, this is not a good thing. I can't speak for all couples, but to my husband it is a simple matter: same = good; different = bad. He really disliked not knowing who would be greeting him at the end of the day: the business-as-usual wife who required little emotional maintenance, or the hypersensitive, agenda-carrying pregnant woman who had moved into his home. Many were the days that he came home to find me poised to land on his head like a tiger crouching in a tree. Perhaps I wanted him to help me assemble the crib, *right then, before he went to the bathroom.* Other times I wanted him to get right back into his car and go out to buy me frozen yogurt. But the times he dreaded the most were conversations that began "You have no idea what it is like to be pregnant. You don't know what I am going through."

He agreed with the premise, but he loathed the conversation, because he knew that I wouldn't feel satisfied until I made him sit and listen to all of my current concerns and dissatisfactions: He wasn't reading the pregnancy books I'd bought for him, he never told me anymore I looked sexy, I was worried that I was too selfish to be a good mother and needed him to tell me I was really the most generous and caring person he had ever known, and so on and so on. By gosh, he *would* know what I was going through, or I would kill both of us trying to explain it.

Normally, when an otherwise happy couple is going through a bumpy time, sitting down and talking out the problem can be quite helpful. This is not true, however, when the better half of the couple is pregnant. Simple biology will preclude the man and woman from having any clue as to what the other is feeling or thinking, and by the end of the nine (ten) months, neither of you will honestly be able to say that you care that much. But don't worry too much, because this communication gap will disappear after the baby is born and you are both physically and emotionally recovered. Parenting is a much more collaborative effort than pregnancy and the two of you will be more in sync with your worries and your joys—equal partners in the "How in the world do we raise a child?" quandary.

You may, one desperate day, find yourself asking your mate point-blank if he thinks you are acting crazy. *This is an utter waste of time.* Any guy with any sort of survival instinct has learned early on to tell you only what you seem to want to hear; in other words, *he will lie.* I know that men lie about these things, because I have interviewed them with their mates *and* alone or with other guys. When they are with their lady, they applaud what a trouper the woman has been during this ordeal, how beautiful and motherly she is becoming, and how much they admire her. Take the lady out of earshot (and throwing distance), and boy oh boy does the tune change. Especially when they are egged on by other partners of pregnant women, these put-upon fellows really let fly. Their mates are schizophrenic, they are constantly whimpering over some imagined slight, they sleep all the time, they eat all the time, they are bitchy. These venting guys finally drive their point home with this boneheaded remark: "I don't know what the big deal is, anyway. My mother had five kids and no car, let alone a cleaning lady, and she didn't lose *her* mind." I know, these are fighting words—but *don't* rise to the occasion.

Pregnancy, to many men, is just not a big enough deal to create such emotional chaos. They simply do not get it. My Girlfriend Maryann's husband is a trained medical man and might be expected to know better, but he devoutly believes that his mate has suffered a nervous breakdown that has *coincidentally* occurred during the first five months of her pregnancy. Nothing anyone says can convince him that her behavior is simply a reaction to the physical and emotional changes that she is going through. That she is pregnant could not *possibly* be significant enough to explain her emotional fragility or her voracious appetites for everything from food to sex. It must be a brain tumor or mental illness.

All of these fellows have horror stories. One tells about a partner who stayed in bed in her pajamas all day. Another describes how his mate threatened a waiter's life at her favorite restaurant when he told her that they were out of popovers. Then there is always some story about a woman who comes home sobbing because the gas station attendant failed to clean her windshield or another driver pulled ahead of her in her lane, or somebody smoked a cigarette near her. (This last bit is a recurring theme: Pregnant women are deeply wounded by people who do not acknowledge their special status by treating them gingerly. They don't ask to be relieved of their regular obligations and responsibilities; they just want a little respect while they are performing them pregnant.)

Naturally, there are exceptions to this description of pregnant partners. For every ten men I give you who feel that it's best to take the defensive position throughout their mate's pregnancy, you will give me one who has never felt more closely bound to his partner than during her pregnancy. We have all heard the myth about the exceptional man who says that his mate's pregnancy is *their* pregnancy, and that he wants to share as much of it with her as he can. This is the guy who not only accompanies his mate to her monthly doctor's visit, but also brings a video camera to the checkup. Personally, I have to wonder about these guys. Does it seem to you that maybe they have too much time on their hands? I don't know, I'm just asking.

A minor drawback of having such an enthusiastic mate is that he might tend to *physically* experience your pregnancy, in addition to identifying with your emotional experience. This can lead to something strange called the couvade syndrome, which is just a pretentious way of saying that the guy gets fat, emotional, and nauseous along with the pregnant partner. I find this loathsome because if your fella is developing symptoms of his own, then before you know it, you will be called on to cater to *him*. Just as when you and your partner both have colds, he always manages to be sicker than you are, now he can be more pregnant than you are. Tell him to go to work and mind his own business.

My husband is a bad comparison because he hated nearly all the activities associated with pregnancy and having babies. (He just liked being a father, and if our babies could have been ordered online, he would have been deeply grateful.) First of all, as a general rule, he gets resentful if anyone in the house is in need of more care than he is. So if I was nauseous, he had food poisoning. If I had bleeding during pregnancy, he was convinced he was developing an ulcer or a heart condition. Second, he is terrified of nearly everything having to do with bodily functions. It still offends him, after countless years of togetherness, when I try to pee and carry on a conversation with him at the same time. This being the case, you can imagine how he felt about coming with me to a vaginal exam.

He also used to be timid about the baby's and my well-being during pregnancy. He got frightened when I would put his hand on my stomach toward the end of my pregnancy to feel the baby do somersaults, when the flips were particularly dramatic. He was convinced that someone was going to get hurt, and that it was my job as the mother to stop all this roughhousing. When I went into labor, he invariably fell asleep (or more accurately, he went unconscious), no matter what time of day or night, because the stress of watching me in any sort of discomfort made him miserable. The only thing that he hated more than cutting the umbilical cord was coming with me to shop for the baby's clothes or furniture. Strolling through a baby store and comparing the musical tunes on various mobiles was like being stuck in a circle of Hades, as far as he was concerned. (Then again, shopping was overwhelming to most parents-to-be I talked to; who in the world knows whether a changing table should be its own piece of furniture or if it should come as part of the bureau?) But once those kids were here and I had survived, my husband became Superdad. So don't worry if your mate's paternal instinct isn't evident yet; it will come.

Mates as Birth Coaches

Almost every couple expecting their first child will enroll in some sort of childbirth-preparedness course. They are motivated by two things: Everybody else has done it, and their obstetrician told them to do it. Most women who are pregnant with their first baby truly hope that a Lamaze or

Bradley class will help them forgo drugs during labor and delivery, or at least help them through the part before they get the drugs. Their partners generally just acquiesce, because long ago they gave up challenging or disagreeing with anything their pregnant partner wanted. Almost 90 percent of the baby daddies I have talked to believe that childbirth-preparedness courses are mandatory, initially looking on this training as a way to finally participate in this experience that heretofore their lady had been hogging. They generally didn't once consider shirking this commitment—until about fifteen minutes into the first class.

When asked, in retrospect, what they thought of their childbirth classes, my Girlfriends' partners almost unanimously rolled their eyes. Sure, they learned many things they hadn't known before, and yeah, the classes might have been a little helpful. But did they *like* them? No. First of all, men in Lamaze classes don't bond as women do. They don't feel particularly close to these strangers simply because they have pregnancy in common, even if their mates have memorized one another's phone numbers and pregnancy histories after the first class. The movies of actual births either scared them or sickened them, and they didn't particularly enjoy seeing a room of fat women, their partner included, lying on their sides and spreading their legs apart in pretend pushing exercises. They even hated walking from the parking lot to the classroom with a bed pillow under their arm as if they were on their way to a slumber party.

Cruel as it may seem, the most universal complaints about childbirth classes were about the *teachers*. I don't know what it is about these women, and I certainly don't want to indict an entire profession, but some *are* a bit strange. I took childbirth-preparedness courses with two of my pregnancies, and neither of my instructors was even in a serious relationship, let alone a mother. My first teacher was particularly reverential about birthing, and she described labor as a sort of touchy-feely lovefest that my husband and I would share. I think she envisioned us both naked and sweaty, with my husband massaging and soothing me through the difficult times. If she had ever given birth herself, she would have known that a husband who touches his wife while she is laboring risks getting his hand bitten—possibly off.

Our second course was a private one taught in our home over a few evenings toward the end of my pregnancy. By the second evening, my husband was so openly hostile to the flower-child instructor that he would get up in the middle of her lecture, order Chinese food over the phone, then eat the whole meal in front of her, without offering her so much as a fortune cookie. When she suggested we watch some videos of other births, he glared at her for trying to ruin his appetite. He actually offered to pay double her class fee if she would agree to sign our "graduation" certificate and not come again.

I am going to go out on a limb here, but here goes: I feel that the current fashionable thinking about the daddy seeing the mommy through the ordeal of delivering a baby is unnecessarily strict and limiting. Don't get me wrong; I think any man who is willing should be there for the labor and delivery—especially the delivery, because it is one of life's undisputed miracles. I also think that all delivering women should consider inviting along another *woman*. One who has had a baby herself is preferable, but any empathetic Girlfriend will do. You might be fortunate and find that your labor and delivery nurse at the hospital fulfills your emotional needs; these women are truly great and can become instant Girlfriends in one's time of need.

With larger birthing rooms all the rage these days, there is usually plenty of room for you, your mate, your doctor, your nurse, and a friend or two. Especially if your labor lasts more than three or four hours—which I can practically guarantee it will—you will find that the companionship of someone other than the guy who got you into all this trouble in the first place will be welcome. Not only will *you* appreciate the companionship of a Girlfriend, but your mate will probably be secretly grateful for the chance to sit down outside somewhere and take a break.

Guys Have Fears of Their Own

Not that I am suggesting it is your job to do anything about it, but it might be nice to occasionally remind yourself that you are not the only one who is turning into a parent in the foreseeable future. You are not the only one in your house with worries and concerns. Daddies have fears of their own, and what follows is a list of most of them, in no particular order.

1. If He Becomes a Father, He Cannot Be the Baby Anymore
A lot of us are with men who require some mothering to keep them happy. They like being nurtured and coddled, and they worry, with good reason, that you will have less time to do this for them if you are doing it

for the baby. As my husband so succinctly said, "You are like a pie. Every time you get pregnant, my piece of the pie gets smaller."

2. A Baby Is So Expensive That the Family Will Go Broke

Even if you don't go bankrupt immediately, at the very least your mate won't be able to get that flat screen he has always wanted. This money worry is often at the top of the charts for guys, probably because they are traditionally expected to provide for the baby, at least while you are incapacitated, and they don't know if they're up to the job. Even if you are a two-income family and you intend to return to work shortly after delivering, the truth remains, babies *are* expensive, and they only get more expensive as they get older. Most of us have, however, already decided that the financial sacrifices are worth it, or we wouldn't have gotten pregnant in the first place.

3. His Partner Will Get Ugly

Well, maybe that's stated too harshly. Perhaps it is more accurate to suggest that he is afraid of not feeling as sexually aroused by the new and enlarged version of his wife. Or maybe he pictures women who don't get out of their bathrobes or wash their hair often enough when they get pregnant, and he worries that you will be like them.

4. His Partner Will Never Go Back to Her Old Self

Remember, your mate fell in love with a woman who looked a certain way, and pregnancy is going to change that look dramatically. Even men who think that their pregnant wife is sexy or cute occasionally have to wonder whether she will do what it takes to get her old figure back, more or less, or if she will forever be altered. Look at Grace Kelly, Elizabeth Taylor, or other such former beauties. They never again looked as they did in *Father of the Bride* or *Rear Window* after having birthed a few children. (We should all look so *bad,* right?) So it can clearly happen to the best of us.

5. The Rational, Stable Partner He Used to Have Will Be Permanently Replaced by This Sobbing, Sleepy, Impatient, Ravenous, Baby-Obsessed Person Who Has Gas

No matter how much he wants to believe that this whole matter of pregnancy-induced insanity is temporary, he will worry that the old, fun you will never come back. It is so hard for men to imagine the emotional effect pregnancy has on a woman, never having experienced even PMS themselves, that they secretly suspect this moodiness is clear evidence of psychosis. If their friends with kids have told them anything about post-partum depression, then they worry that you will continue to be crazy even after the baby is born.

6. He Will Panic When His Partner Goes into Labor and Be Unable to Find His Way to the Hospital

Just as we have nightmares in which we misplace our babies, guys have all sorts of nightmares about how they will mess up at the Big Moment. Every time they drive you to the hospital, whether for a tour, Lamaze classes, or because you are making them practice, they will imagine trying to make the drive when their brains are rendered useless by terror. But don't worry about your partner forgetting how to get to the hospital, because *you* will remember, and you will be yelling directions at him the whole way.

7. He Will Have to Deliver the Baby Himself

He imagines the car breaking down or a blizzard or some other disaster at the moment you need to get to a hospital, and single-handedly having to deliver the baby. That fear is not totally outside the realm of rationality, because nearly all of us have heard some such story. My brother-in-law was backing the car out of the garage during a January snowstorm in New York to take my sister to the hospital to have her baby. He had the driver's door open so that he could see clearly as he reversed down the slippery driveway. The door caught on a snowdrift and ripped right off the car. Do you think that stopped them from getting to the hospital on time? Not on your life. People are capable of amazing feats when they panic, and driving with no door was not going to get in the way of this delivery's occurring in a medical setting.

8. He Will Faint During Delivery (or Worse Yet, He Will Stay Conscious and Have to Watch the Whole Thing)

I think most men imagine fainting in the delivery room because it is one of those clichés from television and movies. Labor and delivery are not rapid, catch-you-off-guard occurrences, but rather slow and deliberate progressions. Therefore, they are not the kinds of things that make people faint. Vomit, perhaps, but not faint.

9. The Doctor Will Insist That He Cut the Umbilical Cord

Now this, on the other hand, does have some fainting elements to it. For one thing, the cord looks unquestionably like a part of the human biology, and therefore not something that most people are inclined to want to damage in any way. Second, when you cut it, *stuff,* such as blood, can come squirting out. If he doesn't know that in advance, your mate may just have his fainting fear come true. My Girlfriend Dona absolutely forbade her husband to cut her daughter's umbilical cord. Given his mechanical ability, it didn't seem like a good idea. It wasn't all that high on his wish list, either, and he was only too happy to leave the task to professionals.

10. Labor and Delivery Will Hurt His Partner, and He Won't Be Able to Make It Better

This is a common and sweet concern among men. Most of my Girlfriends have told me that the hardest thing for their partner was having to watch the woman he loves suffer. The men don't know what to do to make it better, and they may feel faintly guilty at the passive role they must play. (And if they don't, most laboring wives will see to it that they do.) My own husband used to beg me to ask for an epidural the minute I changed out of my clothes and into a hospital gown. His thinking was "We know this is going to hurt eventually, so do us both a favor and take the drugs now."

11. He Will Never Be Able to Have Sex with You Again

A substantial number of men like to think of breasts and vaginas as being designed for one thing: THEM. Intellectually, they know that these organs will have to be shared with the new baby, but sexually, they don't want to know about it. Many men have wondered if they would ever want to have intercourse with their mate again after seeing a bowling ball come out of her. My Girlfriend Patti never discussed this possibility with her husband; she simply headed the whole thing off at the pass by forbidding him to stand anywhere but at her head during delivery. If her doctor had foolishly offered to move a mirror down there so that both of them could see the baby crowning, she would have risked the seven years' bad luck and broken it over his head.

12. His Partner Will Die and Leave Him with Some Strange Baby

Both men and women admit to having irrational fears about the mother dying in childbirth; the mother is concerned for obvious reasons, and the man fears that, in addition to losing someone he is rather fond of, he will be on his own with the baby. With rare exceptions, men think of tending to newborn babies as women's work, and they have a hard time imagining doing *all* of the caring and nurturing of raising a child. Since this baby is still a stranger to him, and his partner is his family, he also worries that he would resent the baby if it were to hurt her in any way. By the way, because you are probably a mite sensitive at this time in your life, let me remind you: It is almost unheard of in this day and age for women to die in childbirth.

13. He Is Bound to This Woman Forever

When you are married without children, the thought of breaking up can be heartbreaking, but you figure you can make the split somehow and eventually get on with your lives. Once the two of you have children together, however, you are in each other's life in a very real way for decades, whether you want to be or not. Kids are a joint, ongoing project, no matter who else you may fall in love with or how much un-in-love the two of you may someday grow to be. The good news is, children keep you so busy and distracted that you may not even notice if your marriage has gone to pot.

14. He Won't Be as Good a Father as His Father Was

A good father is the stuff from which heroes are created. (A mother, no matter how good or bad, becomes the inspiration for psychiatric therapy later in her children's lives.) If a man admired and loved his father, there is sometimes the fear that he could never do the job as well himself. After all, *he* is merely a thirteen-year-old in a man's body, and *his father* was, well, a FATHER. The truth is, once he has a child of his own, your guy will come to see his father for the human being that he was, as uncertain about, but as devoted to, the job of child-rearing as he himself is now.

15. He Will Be as Bad a Father as His Father Was

This is the real world, and a lot of men grew up with a less-than-ideal father or even no father at all. If your partner wasn't all that enamored of his father's parenting abilities, he may be intimidated about becoming a father himself. There are no books or classes that teach you how to parent properly. If you are lucky, you learn it through emulation of your own parents. That can leave the people who have no role models pretty much up in the air. Or worse, they develop unrealistic expectations for parenthood based on their childhood fantasies of what a *good* daddy would have been like, fantasies based on fairy tales and television-sitcom fathers.

For new fathers, as well as new mothers, *The Girlfriends' Guide*'s advice is to trust your instincts; you will be fine at this parenting business. The biggest part of the job is showing up and loving this baby. If you are present, you can learn the rest along the way. The Girlfriends and I think that this worrying business is the greatest burden of pregnancy. So, daddies-to-be, think of us Girlfriends as *your* support group, too. We can't cure you of worrying, but we will keep you company (and probably make fun of you a little) while you do it.

12

When the Old-Fashioned Way Isn't Working

(Miscarriages, Multiples, Assisted Reproduction, and C-Sections)

IN THE TWELVE years since I first wrote *The Girlfriends' Guide to Pregnancy*, the biggest change has to be in the marriage of chemistry and pregnancy. It's common for couples planning to have children to have ovulation-predictor kits, basal thermometers, and pregnancy kits in the bathroom closet alongside the tampons and the Astroglide. With all these opportunities to know the most auspicious day to make a baby, whether from our psyche, our vaginal mucus, the drop in our basal temperature, or a change in color in our ovulation predictor, even those of us who aren't worried that we can have a baby when we want to can't resist the urge to check it out.

Those of us who have been trying to make a baby for six months to a year with no success often cut right to the chase and try such drugs as Clomid and injections of ovulation-stimulating drugs such as Gonal F and Lupron; not to mention sperm analysis for our mates, sperm "washing" and intrauterine insemination (affectionately known in my house as "turkey basting"); and finally, combining one or more of these techniques with in vitro fertilization (the old "test-tube baby") and occasionally preimplantation genetic testing.

You've Won the Reproductive Lottery; Now Why Can't You Relax?

Since you are reading this book, I'm going to assume that you are, indeed, with child. Sure, lots of Girlfriends who are not pregnant buy this book to give as a gift to one who is, and others page through it and giggle while standing in the bookstore, but experience has shown me that buying this book and reading it cover to cover is a sort of rite of passage for Girlfriends who "qualify" by passing the pregnancy test. Call it superstitious, but those of us who have a hard time getting pregnant and holding it *are* extremely superstitious people.

So you might be asking why I'm even talking about fertility treatments in a book about people who have, by definition, passed or skipped that stuff. I am writing about it because, if you have had a hard time getting pregnant and/or staying pregnant, your experience for the next nine months may be very different from that of those Girlfriends who drank a few too many pomegranate martinis and had a baby forty weeks later. As a woman who had her first baby at the age of thirty-four, after three years of trying and nearly two years of shots, blood tests, ultrasounds, inseminations, prayers, bargains with God, and absolute devastation every time my period started, I know of which I speak.

Miscarriage

My Girlfriend Lara got pregnant right after she started trying. It was kind of a joke because her version of "trying" was to forget if she'd taken her pill that weekend. Everything worked just as it does on TV. She didn't even get nauseous and kept telling the rest of us that she sometimes forgot she was even pregnant. One weekend, about ten weeks after she'd laughingly passed her pregnancy test stick around to all of us at lunch, I called her to see if she wanted to hang with me over the weekend since both our mates were out of town. She didn't call me back on Saturday or Sunday. I just figured she'd gotten a better offer and wrote it off.

Late Sunday night, our Girlfriend Thea called me from Lara's house and whispered that Lara had been experiencing cramps and some bleeding all weekend, and did I think Thea should insist Lara go to the hospital? What did I know? But the severity of the cramping and Lara's frightened tears had them at the OB's first thing the next morning. By the time I got there, Lara had had a D&C and was foggy on Valium. She was also numb with grief.

I got it right then that the *idea* of a baby, the dream of it and having it in your life forever, begins as soon as that baby makes its presence known. The mourning that a mother does when she loses that baby is of the most profound and inconsolable kind. It's primitive and indescribable. And to those who are not the mother, it's baffling and bigger than what they would have expected. The most important thing I can tell those other people is that reassurances like "You'll get pregnant again in no time, so don't let this bother you" or "You know, it's probably best that you lost this one because it must have had something really wrong with it" or "It's nature's way of fixing things" are not only unhelpful, they are deeply hurtful and show ignorance or lack of respect for the love this mother has for this baby.

It's only natural for a woman who has experienced this loss and finds herself pregnant again to feel more anxiety than exhilaration, particularly for the first trimester, when most miscarriages occur. The same goes for a woman such as me, who worked and wanted and hoped for a baby for so long: When I finally got pregnant, the celebration lasted twenty-four hours, and then the worry set in for the next nine months. It's natural for pregnant women to fuss and worry and get finicky and moody, but for some of us, this is a journey that we can't wait to end safely. All you Girlfriends who feel that you'd rather skip all the baby-name books, the shopping for infant uggs, and the announcement to family and friends at Thanksgiving that at this time next year there will be one more for dinner, my Girlfriends Cindy, Rachel, Pam, Mindy, Lara, Susie, and Peggy feel your pain!

And don't you worry about feeling this way or guilty that you're just not in the mood to jump up and down in joyous celebration; first, because you're too anxious, and second, because you don't want to risk jarring the baby from his feeble hold in your uterus and falling out. What you feel is so real and understood by those who've walked a mile in your moccasins. And what you feel today has nothing to do with how you'll feel tomorrow and the next day and the next. Maybe you'll never relax; maybe you will by the time you get your amnio results (although I was so traumatized by realizing that my risk of miscarrying during the test was equal to my risk of having a child with Down syndrome—1 in 200—that I got up off the table with the Betadine still wet and brown on my belly and left the doctor's office sobbing uncontrollably). Perhaps the heartbeat will reassure you. For me, I didn't fully relax until recently, when my first baby graduated high school and got into a good college—but, hey, I'm a victim of my hormones!

After three years of wanting a baby with all my heart and countless agreements with God that I would never complain about stretch marks or projectile vomiting or hemorrhoids if I could just get pregnant, when it finally happened, I whinged and moaned about smells that offended me, sheets that weren't soft enough, a husband who couldn't find food fast enough for my powerful hunger when we were driving on the freeway, and the bed rest that was ultimately prescribed for me. I cannot believe that I thought bed rest was a punishment and took the "fun" out of my pregnancy! I'd trade my spleen and my diamond stud earrings for that doctor's order today. But here's the good news about my little tantrums and fears: My child was born in perfect health and I got through three more pregnancies and my love for all four of them is boundless. You see, God didn't punish me for being a brat, and I know you won't be punished, either. Isn't that a relief?

There's no science in this next bit; actually, there's no real science anywhere in this book, but I digress. . . . It's just that I spent a year researching (in my "Girlfriendish" way, which meant listening to countless Girlfriends who'd been through infertility treatment, and collecting anecdotal information for a book I might write someday) and I've noticed that lots of us who had trouble conceiving had trouble carrying. That's not medical research talking here, Girlfriends, just a personal hunch. My Girlfriend Cindy and I both ended up on bed rest by the middle of our second trimesters. I was allowed to shower for three minutes a day and to get up only to use the toilet. She was put in the hospital until her baby was "cooked." We both ended up having C-sections as soon as our little boys' lungs were strong enough to live outside our wombs.

Call it coincidence, call it modern science allowing us to hold on to pregnancies that might not have made it on their own; all I know is that I had placenta previa (a potential bleeding condition that resulted from the placenta covering my cervix and blocking the baby's exit), and Cindy had a placenta that wanted to tear under stress. Should we have thwarted Mother Nature by holding on to these babies? You bet your ass, Mama! They are two of the most handsome, smart, charming, and spoiled young men on this planet, I'll have you know!

With so many babies being born to us later than the physically optimal age of twenty-four, often with the help of medical treatment, it's natural for some of us to find almost nothing natural about our science fiction pregnancies. We may doubt our abilities to carry children because we weren't able to create them without medical intervention. Plus, those of us who get pregnant with help are often immediately put on progesterone, to help us keep our hormone level high enough to keep the baby—so a positive pregnancy test isn't the finish line, but merely the beginning of a new race. If we hold on to the baby for the first trimester, our fertility doctors may release us from their care to an obstetrician's, but most of us are referred to high-risk OBs and we never forget the category we've been assigned to. If we need high-risk doctors, we must be at high risk of having something bad happen, right? It's like giving your fantasies—about awaking in the middle of the night with a slight twinge in the belly and saying, "Honey, I think it's time," and dashing to the hospital to have a drug-free labor lasting three hours, and a vaginal birth without an episiotomy—a smack over the head with a piece of granite. At least it was for me.

Our Lady of Expectant Mothers, Brooke Shields, should get the Nobel Prize for sharing her experience with postpartum depression, and I will talk more about that very real condition later. But for this chapter, the important details she shared with us were her difficulty in getting pregnant, the hormones she took to make a baby, and the fears she carried throughout her pregnancy. She thinks they were important elements in the painful depression that followed. Uh, yeah! When we've been dreaming about something that we might call our biological imperative and we've got DNA, hormones, societal expectations, and childhoods with Cabbage Patch babies and Betsy Wetsy dolls, then we are told we can't experience it, or only imperfectly, it can be a big drag.

When a woman wants to express herself in the world, to get an education, achieve some experience and wisdom, gain financial security, and—oh, yeah, I almost forgot—find a MAN (or woman—Rosie and Kelli, I love your family) with whom to share a commitment, she may be much older than her midtwenties before getting pregnant. In fact, like the lady in one of my favorite cartoon drawings, she may say with anguish, "Oh my God, I forgot to have kids!"

If we find ourselves in our midthirties or early forties, we may sprint to a reproductive specialist to help us have a baby or two or three, before the curtain falls on our egg factory. We may even use donor eggs from a younger woman to create a pregnancy with our partner. This usually involves in vitro fertilization, which carries the inherent risk of multiple embryos. "Hurrah!" many Girlfriends have shouted when given the prospect of creating a family of four in one IVF pregnancy. It's only later that we learn the risks this new opportunity can present.

Twins, while being a particular delight and gift, are also considered a high-risk pregnancy. The pregnancy can be harder: The morning sickness can be twice as intense, the weight gain can be much greater, the pressure on mom's spine and bladder are double, they can sap her bones dry of any calcium that they want, and so on. The most significant risk is that they are almost always born prematurely. Premature birth can increase many risks for the babies and I don't need to freak us all out with the details. I'm just bringing it up here to give another example of certain pregnancies, which we want more than life itself, not always being full of joy and gratitude. We're allowed to not be grateful at times, Girlfriends!! Go ahead and torment those closest to you when you can't take it another second; these aren't just YOUR pregnancies, they're your mate's, the grandparents', and the whole damn village's that Hillary Clinton keeps talking about.

The Secrets That No One Will Tell

Some "miscarriages" are not spontaneous abortions, as the medical books call them, but rather are the result of searingly painful decisions that the parents must make—usually in such shame or fear of being judged harshly that they carry the burden silently, without the support of their friends and family. The first type occurs when an amniocentesis or CVS (chorionic villus sampling) indicates that the unborn child is genetically defective. The second type occurs more and more with the frequency of multiple embryos and is called selective termination.

Since prenatal genetic testing such as amnio and CVS have been around for quite a while and more mothers-to-be qualify for them by virtue of being over thirty-five, it's become a part of our consciousness that we may actually have to do something if the results are not what we'd hoped. My Girlfriend Danica and her husband finally got pregnant after a couple of miscarriages, and this one was a keeper. Ultrasound showed a heartbeat at nine weeks, and they relaxed into the belief that their dream had finally come true. Danica went in for her amnio, being over thirty-five, and in the meantime, she was starting to get an adorable bump, and we all teased her about finally getting a bustline. One Girlfriend even offered to throw the baby shower.

I don't even need to tell you that the amnio results were bad. A decision had to be made whether to see if Mother Nature would terminate this pregnancy herself or if Danica and Lenny should do so. They eventually chose termination, and never was a decision more agonizingly made. Would it have been better not to know at all? I don't have a clue. All I do know is that the technology that is available now to provide information about the embryo's health can either be immensely reassuring or lead to some horrible decisions about what to do with that information when it's bad.

Doctors performing IVF customarily put as many fertilized eggs as they can back into the mother in forty-eight hours. Some clinics refuse to put more than three embryos back, but no laws prevent the depositing of four or more embryos in most states in the United States. It's not usually that the doctors are stupid or cruel or driven by the desire to keep their pregnancy percentages up for profit motives. Rather, it's their experience that often no embryos become implanted and grow into fetuses. Or they know that the mother's eggs are getting less viable with each IVF cycle, or that she's about to stop the treatment because she can't afford it anymore.

Whatever the motivation, some of my Girlfriends not only got the blessed news that they were going to be mothers after that last IVF round, but that they were going to have twins or even triplets or quadruplets. At least four times a year, our local television news stations announce that some woman has just had five babies, and though they're all incredibly small and several weeks or months premature, the parents are thrilled and staring into the cameras like deer in headlights. I don't know why, but the mothers always seem to be wearing glasses, which brings up this serious consequence of premature and underweight births: The oxygen that such young babies need has to be artificially provided, and a side effect is sometimes blindness or diminished vision. Take a look at the follow-up visits with those large families and count the children wearing thick glasses and you'll see how frequently this occurs.

I recently watched one of those makeover shows in which a mother of quints had lost all her pregnancy weight, but her husband still didn't find her sexually attractive because she had a flap of empty skin about the size of carry-on luggage hanging over her low-rise jeans. The show paid for it to be surgically removed, but I'll bet those quints have a dozen more tricks up their sleeves for putting the wet blanket on those fires of passion. Then again, so do singleton babies, so that must be an occupational hazard of becoming a parent.

The novelty and possibilities of having the dream for a family come true, in spades, may at first glance seem like the answer to all a parent's prayers. One gestation, one ten-month period of inconvenience and discomfort, and the couple can go from being completely childless to having the American Dream of 2.2 kids, statistically speaking. It's exciting and exhilarating and it gets scads of attention from family, friends, and complete strangers, and that feels wonderful after all the disappointments the couple has endured.

The first ones to prick this balloon are the doctors. They know the toll it takes on the babies, the mother, and the lingering effects for both. Most doctors are not ecstatic about twins and are positively unenthusiastic about triplets or more. When the dangers and risks are considered, the doctor will usually present the parents with the option of terminating one or more of the fetuses, so that the strongest one or two can more safely continue to develop in the womb. Talk about too much information. This is Solomon's choice, and no woman (or man, but I don't think they feel it quite so intimately as the mother) outside of the Bible should be asked to make it.

You know what I just heard? I just heard that nearly 50 percent of all kids accepted in private schools in the major metropolitan areas of Los Angeles, New York, Dallas, San Francisco, and Boston in the year 2007 will be the product of assisted reproductive techniques (ART). I can't give you any definitive statistics, but this factoid came up at a RESOLVE meeting I attended last year. RESOLVE is the national support and educational organization for parents who struggle with infertility. If you think I've flipped my wiggy, just check it out yourself. How many fraternal twins can you count in your niece's playgroup? At your high school reunion, how many old friends are pulling out baby pictures with two kids in a side-by-side stroller?

Here's what it looks like at my kids' elementary school: three sets of fraternal twins, usually a boy and a girl, in each class of forty five-year-olds. I don't care how many times stars like Julia Roberts and Geena Davis tell us disingenuously that "twins run in the family." I think it's a safe bet, when the mother is approaching or passing forty and hasn't been reproductively successful in the past five or six years, that she has turned to ART to help her start her family. In vitro fertilization is responsible for most of these multiples, and also for some precious singletons.

Before I come off as judgmental or a hater, let me tell you that I'm one of THEM. Yup, in a black-lit room, the universal sign for Ovulation Stimulating Hormone comes up on my forehead. At the age of thirty, shortly after marrying my sweet, unsuspecting husband, I committed the following year to quasi-stalking him to have "productive sex" (meaning getting busy when there was actually an egg to fertilize). I deceived him about my intentions, preferring to look horny rather than desperate, and he bought it hook, line, and sinker. Men can be so teeny-brained, especially where lots of unencumbered sex is concerned—bless their little hearts.

After a year of getting jiggy with it, we still had no pregnancy to show for it, so I swallowed my pride and left my "regular girls' " obstetrician and skulked to a practice devoted solely to infertile women. It still hurts to admit that I was asking to be a member of a club that was populated with a bunch of people I didn't want to relate to. I think I wore a baseball cap and sunglasses for the first year. Hey, no ego problem here, folks. It was three more years of treatment in this infertility practice before I finally got pregnant. Keep in mind that this was in the dark ages of infertility treatment, but I got pregnant with our first child, a masculine child, as they say in *The Godfather*.

Anyway, after getting shots every day for about a week and ultrasounds to check my follicles for about four to five days, I was finally given an injection of the hormone HCG, which stands for "human chorionic gonadotropin," to release the egg or eggs that were mature.

One Saturday morning, right before I was to hold a press conference for sports reporters, society doyennes, educators, parents, and athletes who were participating in the California State Special Olympics Games, I drove so fast with a sperm sample from my husband held firmly between my thighs that I was stopped on the empty streets of LA by a traffic cop. Call me hormonal and stressed or call me postal; I came within inches of taking the lid off the precious liquid that was nice and toasty between my loving thighs and tossing it right into the face of the cop. But as much as I wanted to mess with his little mind, I wanted still more to protect that little cup of sperm and deliver it to Nurse Connie.

Although you would have thought that my restraint with the police officer would have given me a free karma pass for the rest of the day, I drove right over a stupid pigeon who wasn't used to the fast pace of eating dead stuff from the middle of the street and flying away before a fancy German sedan caught up to him. The moment I saw his lifeless body in the street from my rearview mirror, I realized that I was the last person God would trust with a child.

In pitiful tears, I pulled into the parking lot and dragged myself upstairs to Dr. Danzer's office to reluctantly hand my husband's specimen to Nurse Connie. I wept in disgrace as I said, "They're all dead," and slid down the lab wall in abject hopelessness. "Come look at this," Connie commanded from her position at the microscope. I had no backbone of my own, but Connie scared me, so I always did as she said, and I walked up to the microscope to see for myself the decimation of the potential Iovine population. To my shock, I saw little sperm bumping as if it were salsa night at Carlos and Pepe's. That visual image made me a believer again, and when the cleaned-and-spun-and-placed-into-a-good-swimming-medium sperm were injected into my uterus in a procedure called IUI (intrauterine insemination), a miracle occurred. Our baby boy was conceived. Sure, my intimate moment was shared with Nurse Connie rather than my partner, but, hey, he was peacefully resting (maybe even puffing on a cigarette) and washing off all the baby oil with a warm, wet washcloth. I was sharing the afterglow with Connie and asking how long before I could get up and put my panties on, because I had the *LA Times* waiting for me.

That whole reproductive nightmare left me with two psychotic tendencies: to be extremely superstitious (read, obsessed with rituals and magical thinking) and the secret belief that if something bad happened, it would be my husband's fault because:

A. He didn't do the rituals I prescribed with proper conviction, if at all.
B. He didn't concentrate on the pregnancy every minute of every day.
C. He didn't treat me like the precious vessel that I was. In fact, he seemed nervous and afraid in my presence.

Just between us Girlfriends, after nearly twenty years, I still don't think I can forgive him, but don't tell him I told you.

Zipper Deliveries

Cesarean section deliveries are becoming almost as frequent as vaginal deliveries in many parts of this country, even when Girlfriends from this country go to, oh, say, AFRICA to have their baby. The reasons are said to range from the convenience of the delivering doctor, to the lowered risk of malpractice claims against your HMO, to the fear of damaging the girly parts, to the ability to get a tummy tuck at the same time, to the need for a Girlfriend to feel in control of something after this dizzying nine (ten) months with the Body Snatcher living inside her.

I think that it's important to add multiple births to that Mad Hatter's list of reasons. There aren't that many doctors these days who will blithely sit by while a mommy of twins or more tries to keep up her hee-hee breathing long enough to wait for each baby to line up in an orderly fashion and exit the mother ship. First, time is money. Second, chances are that these babies are premature and more fragile than full-term singletons and can't take a moment of oxygen deprivation or stress. Heck, under those circumstances, even I would go in after those little dollies.

My first baby, the one we call Pu Yi, after the last emperor of China, the most holy and precious baby ever born to this world, the one I conceived with Nurse Connie, was delivered by a scheduled C-section. Of course he was. Part of what I believe was his whole "Hello, I must be going" attitude from conception to birth included nearly falling out of my uterus before implantation finally broke his free fall just above my cervix. It was my fervent insistence that fertility drugs and progesterone and all the rest keep him up in there that created my condition of placenta previa. And then, of course, when it was time for him to come out and own up to all the trouble he'd caused, we had to go in after him. Even though he was delivered four weeks early, by that point it was him or me. I chose him, but my doctor chose both of us, bless his heart.

Delivery Grief

After that wild ride of getting a child, I was numb about vaginal versus cesarean deliveries. I never even tried to do the Lamaze breathing because all that huffing and puffing was never going to be an option for me. Later I felt as if I'd been gypped. I was nature's victim, and my entire experience, I thought, was felt secondhand via specialists and technicians. I was a host body, not a mommy; the people in scrubs put the baby in, cooked the baby, and pulled the baby out.

I felt so robbed of something my soul yearned for that I sought out a new OB when I got pregnant again (the old-fashioned way—go figure). I searched for a doctor who encouraged VBAC (Vaginal Birth After Cesarean) deliveries and found the handsome Dr. Crane, who delivered my next three babies that way. Truth be told, by the time I was pregnant with our last baby, I asked him if he would consider delivering her C-section. He looked at me as if I were the sociopath that he'd long suspected, but I explained that I had tried it both ways and ultimately found them equally satisfying.

I was mostly concerned with whether I would finally get so stretched out down there that my uterus would one day fall out and splat onto the sidewalk while I was waiting for a child to get off the school bus. When he solemnly looked into my eyes and said, "Vicki, the damage was done with the first vaginal, so it won't really make much of a difference," I shuffled out of his office and said I'd see him when my water broke. Just in the nick of time, one of my more candid Girlfriends told me about a slightly more "thorough" kind of repair than the traditional "extra stitch" docs routinely do, which I could request or else schedule with a specialist. It was only for this nip/tuck that I even got an epidural, because I sneezed that little darlin' out.

Getting back to the grief, however; my Girlfriends Maria and Mindy both prepared for childbirth with conviction. They didn't just want a vaginal birth, they wanted to do it drug-free. (This was way back, before anyone listened to me or thought I might know a thing or two about this pregnancy business.) Both of them labored for more than twenty hours. They were in the kind of pain that only fear and no end in sight can create. Their partners were alternately sympathetic, running for an anesthesiologist, and trying to keep the girls true to their naive promises to labor on, no matter what. I call these husbands Golden Retrievers because they continue to act sweet, loyal, and dumb even when all evidence is making it abundantly clear that everyone in their little family had been unimaginative in how big and long and scary the pain of birth can be. The mom is half out of her mind and begging for drugs, and these guys are asking inane questions like "Can't you focus on your Precious Object just a little longer?" Those guys are lucky they don't end up with those Precious Objects jammed down their throats or through their hearts . . . at least.

Finally, it was the insistence of their doctors that got the laboring moms and their clueless husbands to surrender and release their stressed babies via the zipper. Both Maria and Mindy felt like failures when the greatest moments of their lives occurred. Their babies were delivered by C-sections and were scandalously healthy and robust, but the mommies were crushingly exhausted and disappointed. In one case, time eventually healed the trauma and grief, and in the other, subsequent successful vaginal births erased the memory. You want to talk about a recipe for postpartum depression . . .

Women who have unplanned C-sections almost always have some feeling that someone took their birth experience away from them against their wishes. Sometimes they feel that their doctor or mate didn't have faith in them to endure their labor and find the strength to deliver vaginally. Sometimes they blame themselves for being weak and out of control. And almost always, they feel as if the decision was made and the next thing they knew, their surgery was under way. It wasn't about pain, but rather the fear, the high-stakes drama, and that they no longer felt in control of this birth. For a couple of years my Girlfriend Amy couldn't watch the video of her labor and sudden fetal distress leading to a speedy C-section. She wept and felt panicky and slightly victimized when she tried to view it with me.

I don't know when the myth of the thin, athletic, sunny, ambitious, organic, and self-sacrificing woman became part of our culture, but it surely happened in my reproductive era. My mother and her friends looked at me like a freak when I shared my convictions about motherhood done right, but now I think they were a little bit right. Sure, I'm glad I never followed their advice to smoke to keep my weight down or to eat as much tuna and sea bass as I wanted, but I could have been easier on myself, especially where my own sanity was concerned, when it came to pregnancy, delivery, and motherhood.

Buying into the Myth of the Perfect Mother is as much an illness as bulimia, anorexia, or cutting, if you ask me. I don't know when we bought into the conspiracy that we could have it all, all the time. And I don't know how we joined the army of self-sacrificers. But we have, and it's a sin. Since we are the ones who accepted this nonsense, we are the only ones who can kick it to the curb. Girlfriends, this might not seem relevant to you for several more years, but it is my job as your older sister to share this with you—you can do with it what you want.

Having babies may be as natural as the sun rising in the east, but it's still a miracle every time it happens. If you feel anxious at times, it's just your humility acknowledging that having a dream come true is a blessing, not a right. And when yours does come true, you will appreciate it that much more.

13

Coming into the Homestretch

I CAN HONESTLY say that I have never met a woman who, within a month of her due date, wasn't ready to end this maternity marathon. (With the exception of my Girlfriend Mindy, but she was undergoing house repairs as part of her nesting instinct and wasn't sure if there would be a floor to walk on by her due date.) No matter how chipper and enthusiastic they might have been for the preceding eight (nine) months, even the best of them get cranky and impatient. And who can blame them? They can hardly breathe anymore, they have grown too large for all but their biggest clothes, they aren't sleeping well, they have chronic heartburn and indigestion, and they are keenly aware that somehow, someway, that baby is going to have to come out of their bodies, *soon*! They have also usually come to realize that it is easier to care for a baby that is inside you than one that is outside.

There isn't really much to do at this point. Presumably, you will have had your baby shower. You will also have completed your childbirth-preparedness classes. And aside from putting your shower gifts away, your baby's room is probably pretty much organized, or purchased and awaiting delivery. If you have been working outside the home, chances are you have begun your maternity leave or will be doing so soon. You may find that you have the unfamiliar sensation of having time on your hands, time that you fill with alternating bouts of boredom, excitement, and fear.

As if all this anticipation weren't enough to keep you agitated, you will be increasingly irritated by the well-intentioned comments of nearly every person you brush by. They will say things like "Wow! You're *huge*! When is that baby going to be born?" Or every week, when you go to get a manicure or to do your grocery shopping, the clerk will say, "You mean you *still* haven't had that baby?" Your mother and mother-in-law will call you every single day on the pretense it's just a chat, but really to see if you are in labor and have neglected to tell them. Talk about the watched pot never boiling. . . .

In this chapter we will offer a laundry list of the physical and emotional adjustments required to survive the last month of pregnancy. This may seem like the longest yard, but if you want to be reminded that you are almost finished, look ahead to the next chapter: It's about going to the hospital.

"I Can't Breathe!"

If you are under five feet nine inches and have a normal-sized baby growing inside you, just the act of filling your lungs will become difficult, if not impossible. The placenta—the space bubble that your baby is living in—grows upward and eventually pushes against your diaphragm and your lungs. At this point most babies are head down in the blastoff position, so it is their bottoms and feet that are doing much of the encroaching. Call me crazy, but I found this breathing difficulty alarming. I tend to be a bit claustrophobic anyway, and this gentle suffocating sensation really bugged me. I would stand as tall as I could, fold my arms under my breasts, and pull up, as if I could create more space in there for the baby and me.

The best thing you can do at this stage of your pregnancy is to get on the floor on your hands and knees. This allows gravity to pull the baby forward and away from your spine and organs. It feels so good, you will wish you could crawl through the rest of your pregnancy. This is also a good position to try during labor, for a change of pace. Another reason why you will find yourself huffing and puffing more than The Little Engine That Could at the end of your pregnancy is from the sheer physical exertion of carrying around thirty or forty extra pounds.

An additional pregnancy condition that can cause breathing problems is "pregnancy rhinitis," which is a chronic stuffy nose. Because the inside of your nose is lined with the same soft membrane that lines your vagina, it tends to succumb to the swelling that your vagina experiences. While full vaginal walls and labia can be sexually arousing, full sinus passages are merely heavy breathing without the fun. The miracle about this irritating condition is that it disappears almost the instant the baby is born. Until then, there isn't much you can do about it but sniffle.

"I Can't Eat Any More!"

Just as the growing baby has crowded your lungs and diaphragm, your stomach gets smashed flat like a pancake. You can no longer eat very much at one sitting because there isn't room in there for more than a few bites. You might think that this is welcome news, but don't get too excited, because it doesn't translate into any measurable weight loss. This is probably because you eat less at each meal, but you eat a lot more meals. By this point, what else is there to do? Some of the Girlfriends have reported that they have lost a couple of pounds right before labor, but not usually over the entire last month.

Another physical condition that may lessen your enthusiasm for those hearty meals that characterized your middle trimester is indigestion. Those less fortunate of us may have experienced heartburn and rumbling tummies for much of our pregnancy, but at the end this condition can become much more pronounced. By this time, your baby's behind is so vigorously pressing against your diaphragm that your esophagus is stressing out and not keeping your food down in your stomach, where it belongs. You may be back to eating the comfort foods of early pregnancy—unless, of course, you are gambling that the old wives' tales are true, and that spicy foods do indeed help bring on labor. No matter what you eat, antacids are the perfect dessert.

"I Can't Sleep!"

Being unable to go to sleep and stay asleep were my greatest challenges at the end of my pregnancies. Being tired was no guarantee that I was going to snooze when I went to bed each night. Some Stepford Wives cheerfully told me that this was nature's way of preparing me for the sleepless nights that I would experience as a new mother. That's like saying dieting will prepare you for starvation! As far as I was concerned, a nature that was capable of giving chameleons the gift of disguise wouldn't be stupid enough to think that the cure for no sleep was *more* no sleep.

No, you can't sleep for two major reasons. First, the baby is pulling or sitting on every part of your body but your face and your feet (and those are swollen from water retention). Second, you are so preoccupied with what lies ahead—labor, delivery, *motherhood*—that you have a hard time turning your brain off at night. (Which is kind of ironic, because you will swear that you haven't been able to turn your brain *on* most days.)

Now is the time to reappraise your relationship with your bed pillows. They will grow to become your best friends—not only the one or two that you have always known and loved, but all the new pillows you will buy (or steal from your husband) to help them in their duties. The Girlfriends and I agree that you will need at least three pillows by this point: one between your knees to keep your hips supported (I will explain why that works later), one propped slightly under your pregnant belly, and one under your head and shoulders. Even better, you should consider buying one of those full-length body pillows that are sold in a million catalogs these days. I bought one, and after I got over the shock of how very big it was, I gamely brought it into bed. It felt magnificent, but it created a barrier between my husband and me that would have required helium to ascend. My husband referred to my giant pillow as my "boyfriend," and I actually named it Phil. Fortunately, or unfortunately, depending on my mood, my husband wasn't finding me particularly irresistible, so he never complained about the Great Wall of China between us. I think he might have been grateful.

The one difficulty about my relationship with Phil was when I wanted to turn over. First I would prepare to hurl myself from one side to the other, then I would grab Phil with both arms and both legs and flip it over with me like an alligator wrestler. It invariably shook the bed so violently that my husband nearly fell out, and the comforter would land somewhere halfway across the room.

I am afraid we don't have nearly as good or specific advice for making our brain comfortable enough to sleep. Your doctor may put me on *America's Most Wanted* for saying this, but I think that women who are coming to the end of a healthy and uneventful pregnancy deserve an occasional glass of wine before bed. A little toddy, along with a hot bath (not too hot, of course), can work wonders on the anxious insomniacs that most mothers-to-be become. Ask your doctor first, of course. Maybe I'm just a wino-in-waiting.

One of the biggest culprits in the pregnancy insomnia crisis is the tendency to get leg cramps. I have no idea why we get them, but I do know that they are incredibly common. One minute you are clinging to your body pillow and dreaming about sex with some stranger, and the next you are doubled over in a frantic attempt to massage out a muscle that has contracted like a snapped rubber band. Stretching my lower legs and flexing my feet could make my calf muscle spasm so violently that I thought my Achilles tendon was being removed without anesthesia. My only advice is to walk it off; there is really nothing else to be done.

"I Can't Walk!"

Everybody knows that you can recognize a pregnant woman from behind, whether you can see her big belly or not. The first giveaway is usually her choice of shoes; they are large and roomy and definitely flat. In fact, they may even be scuffs or house slippers if the woman is beyond caring anymore. The poor dear's extremities may be retaining so much water that nothing else fits. Her feet, in these big, shapeless shoes, drag and shuffle between steps, creating a locomotive sound. These feet are generally not within shouting distance of each other, with one supporting one hipbone and the other about three feet away, supporting the other. Topping this all off is the traditional swayback of the very pregnant woman, where she looks as though she is pushing her belly ahead of her in a wheelbarrow.

Before I ever got pregnant, I looked contemptuously upon these slouching, scuffling women, wondering how low their self-esteem had to be to allow them to present themselves to the world in this condition. The least they could do, I thought with indignation, was to keep their legs together when they sat down. My mother, she who weighed all of 120 pounds at her most pregnant, would tsk-tsk behind these struggling souls and whisper to me that if I ever let myself go like that when I got pregnant, she wouldn't be seen in public with me.

Well, I did let myself go to a certain extent, and by that time I didn't care or notice *who* was seen in public with me. If my mother thought I was going to struggle to look good for her when I didn't even do it for my husband, she had another think coming. At this point, the only person I could still pull myself together for was my obstetrician. I looked like Miss Maternity USA when I went in for my checkups: legs and pits freshly shaved, perfume, high-heeled shoes, clean hair (curled, even), and a tasteful amount of makeup. I felt that if I couldn't pull it together for at least one hour a month, all self-respect was truly lost. After the appointment, I would hurry home to change into something huge and stretchy and pig out.

One reason I was able to look decent in the doctor's office was because he never had to see me walk very far. If he had, he would have seen that I could no longer bring my knees together, and that my hip joints were so loose that I felt as though my thighbones would pop out of the sockets with every step. Imagine that your bones are held in their proper positions by elastic bands. In pregnancy, these bands relax to allow your bones to spread apart to accommodate the pregnancy and eventual birth. As I mentioned earlier, your rib cage actually widens to allow for the pregnancy to spread up into that region. And I am sure you will be happy to hear that your pelvis spreads apart, too, to allow for the little watermelon to make its way out. (This is when a "Phil" pillow becomes essential.) So I guess you could call this ligament loosening a good thing.

But it is also a troublesome thing if you jump out of bed in the middle of the night to pee and fall immediately to the floor because your legs slipped out of the standing/walking position. I remember feeling as if I had stepped into a hole, so awkward was my balance and so asymmetrically did my legs settle in their hip joints. If you have dreamed of doing splits again for the first time since your cheerleader days, this may be your chance, because you will be pretty flexible. The only problem is, once you get all the way down there, who is going to lift you back up? If left to your own devices, you would stay in the split until the baby crowned and knocked you off-balance.

So far, I have described reasons why walking is nearly impossible. Even if you were not pregnant, these biological changes would nearly cripple you. Let's add that you are now housing a full-term baby in your belly, and all the water and placental yuck that comes with the package. And, if this is your first baby, it either has already or will soon drop lower into the pelvis in preparation for birth. This dropping—or "lightening," as it is sometimes called—does wonders for your breathing, because it moves the baby away from your diaphragm, but it makes walking an even crueler joke. Do you remember those childhood contests where you held a balloon between your knees and raced across a field? Being nine (ten) months pregnant with a baby that has dropped can feel something like that. Except now they're *water* balloons.

Speaking of a baby dangling between your thighs, my Girlfriend Colleen has coined the quaint term *vagina farts* for the squishy noises that sometimes emanate from between your legs when your baby is low and pressing hard on your cervix and the surrounding area. You can sometimes sound like a whoopee cushion when you walk.

Returning to your weight gain for a second, the last factor to consider in your inability to stride or slink in your former way is the thirty to forty pounds of fat, water, and baby that upholster your body. All overweight people waddle a bit, even without their ligaments being fully released and without a baby's head threatening to protrude between their legs. You don't run to catch the phone anymore, you couldn't jump for a million dollars, and you lose your balance just getting out of the car. I cannot tell you how many of my Girlfriends have reported falling flat on their face during the last few weeks of pregnancy. The good news is, the babies are never any worse for the trauma.

"My Back Hurts!"

If there is any way to treat yourself to a massage toward the end of your pregnancy, please do so. Ask around of other mothers, nurses, or child-birth-preparedness instructors, because they might know of a masseuse who's familiar with the aches and pains of a very pregnant woman. There are even massage tables with pop-out centers so that you can lie on your stomach and have your baby comfortably nestled in a sort of pouch. I thought that this was the most wonderful thing, because I really started to yearn to sleep on my stomach after about six months of being on my side. One last thing: There are certain delicacies about the very pregnant body that only another woman can understand, so no matter how open-minded you might be about getting massages from men when you are not pregnant, when you are pregnant, insist upon a woman.

By the way, all of the pregnancy books that I have read over the years suggested that the baby daddies learn massage and counterpressure techniques to help their mates get through pregnancy and delivery. It always looked so intimate and sweet in the books, but I don't know of one single Girlfriend who was ever cosseted through maternity in this way. One night when I was desperate, I begged my husband to massage my lower spine. He was so unimaginative in his massaging that he never moved his fingers from one single position, and I ended up with something resembling a rug burn on my back. My Girlfriends unanimously reported that when their partners feebly tried to rub them during labor, they screamed at them, "Get your hands off me!" (More about not wanting to be touched during labor in chapter 15.)

It is easy to see why women get all sorts of aches and pains in their spines. The weight of your belly is concentrated within an area that is only about a foot long, and this can seriously pull your spine forward, thereby forcing you to hold your upper back unnaturally far back to compensate for the forward drag. Also, if your breasts are particularly heavy, they can pull on your shoulders and upper back. The best relief that we can suggest is to rest for a while on your left side with a Phil pillow between your legs and under your head and shoulders. (The left side is the medically recommended side because it allows for the most unimpeded flow of blood from your heart to your legs and baby.) You can also try the hands and knees back stretches I described earlier. Or you can sit cross-legged on the floor (what we used to call Indian style in elementary school). This cross-legged sit lets your belly rest on your calves and off your spine. If all of this fails to bring you any relief, call your doctor and ask if you can take an over-the-counter pain reliever.

"I Am Getting So Big That I Might Explode!"

By about the eighth (ninth) month of pregnancy, most first-timers mistakenly believe that their bellies cannot possibly get much bigger. They are as round as if they had swallowed a basketball, their skin is stretched, and all the clothes in the maternity stores fit them perfectly. And then come the last four weeks. . . .

The pregnant belly of a woman who is about to give birth is not a graceful, rounded belly, but rather a thin covering of skin stretched over a child's elbows, knees, and bony bottom. I always say that you can tell a woman is finishing her pregnancy when her stomach develops "corners." The baby is now so big and strong that at times its body parts are most definitely recognizable to your touch and seemingly recognizable to your eye. If your tummy isn't oddly shaped and threatening to rupture your belly button, your baby probably isn't cooked enough yet. Think of yourself as a Butterball turkey—when your belly button pops out, you're about done.

"My Doctor Says I Could Go into Labor at Any Minute!"

As you come into the homestretch, you will begin to see your obstetrician more frequently, first every two weeks, then every week for the last three or four weeks. You may have noticed earlier that your doctor seldom, if ever, performed a vaginal exam once the pregnancy was established. Now he or she will start peeking up inside you again to look for some of the signs that birth is imminent.

Your doctor will begin to give you reports like "You are fifty percent effaced and one centimeter dilated." (*Effacement* and *dilation* refer to the cervix getting ready to let the baby out. More about these phenomena in chapters 15 and 16.) You will leave the office filled with anxiety, certain that you are going into labor that night, if you even make it through dinner. You will call your friends and relatives and put them on red alert in preparation for the call that you are in labor. When the baby still hasn't come three days later, you start looking forward to your next doctor's visit to hear more about effacement and dilation. I don't know why, but we all grasp on to this information as if it meant something, and it doesn't really mean much at all. The world is filled with women who live for weeks 70 percent effaced and three centimeters dilated. There are just as many women who go home after being told by their doctors that they are still closed tight as a drum, only to have their water break during dinner and their babies born before breakfast.

I could spend the next twenty pages telling you not to set too much store by these measurements, and you would still ignore me. Just as earlier in this *Girlfriends' Guide* I warned you not to count on your due date as an exact indication of when to expect your baby and you ignored me, you will wish me wrong on this matter. I know, because I did the same thing.

"I Can't Take One More Day of This!"

There will come a time, when you have about forty weeks under your belt (literally), that you start listening to folk wisdom about how to bring on labor and get this show on the road. I am treading on thin ice here, but I would be foolish if I pretended that you haven't heard about any of these things and haven't considered trying them. You know what I'm talking about: Going on a long walk, having vigorous sex, eating hot, spicy food, drinking cod-liver oil, and giving yourself an enema are all "home remedies" for "curing" a never-ending pregnancy. There was even a Hollywood restaurant that served a garden salad that was rumored to bring on labor. For a couple of weeks it became a story on the local news programs. Doctors and scientists studied the piles of lettuce and other grassy ingredients, only to give varying reports as to which was the magic potion. Some thought that it could be the cilantro (an herb used in a lot of Mexican and Chinese food). Others suggested that the exotic balsamic vinegar used to make the dressing was causing all the contractions. Either way, on any given day you could go for lunch at this restaurant and find several ripely pregnant women eating salad with gusto.

Of all the ways to encourage your labor to step it up a bit, walking is the most popular among doctors and fitness fanatics. I myself found an intravenous drip of pitocin to be slightly more effective, but you already know about my desire to cut to the chase in these matters. I did commit to a walking regimen with three of my pregnancies, because I was willing to try anything to get things moving along. I walked in deep sand on the beach, I race-walked through shopping malls (I must have looked like a clipper ship at full sail), and I insisted on taking stairs instead of elevators whenever possible. Sad to say, not once did any of my babies take the hint and consider moving out. Things were different after my water broke, however, and that walking business was suddenly a lot more effective. In fact, I had just enough time to stroll around the block a couple of times before I had contractions measurable enough to get the hospital to give me a labor room.

I must seriously tell you that once your water has broken, the baby will probably be born within a matter of a few hours, or else risk of infection might develop as its pristine little bubble becomes exposed. *Always* call your doctor if you think that you have sprung a leak or that you are urinating uncontrollably. In fact, if your due date (myth though it may be) comes and goes without any unique event, your doctor may consider moving things along by breaking your water for you. By the time the due date for my fourth baby arrived, I think I would have tried to pop my own bag of waters if my arm had been long enough. But as they say on TV, "Do not attempt this stunt at home. It should only be performed by trained professionals."

My Girlfriend Caroline swears that vigorous sex at the end of pregnancy will bring on labor. From what I have read, some science actually supports this notion, something about semen having a chemical like pitocin. I also think that "massaging" the cervix with penetration of your mate's you-know-what helps wake it up after nine (ten) months of sleeping and prepares it to stretch open. Then again, Caroline is well-known for her insatiable lust, so maybe this was just her ploy to get her husband to consent to mercy sex when he would have preferred to watch the second half of *Monday Night Football.*

A technique that used to be called "stripping the membrane" is now more euphemistically called "performing a vigorous internal examination." It is, of course, done by your doctor, and only after he or she is fully satisfied that the baby is completely baked and ready to pop out of the oven. I guess this technique works along the same lines as vigorous sex, but without the fun, in giving a wake-up call to your cervix. If you and your doctor agree to do this, be prepared for it to hurt like bad menstrual cramps and to be accompanied by as much blood as the beginning of your period. This "vigorous exam" may accomplish absolutely nothing (it never got my contractions to start), but I am told you stand a better chance of going into labor if the cramping sensation persists for a few hours, rather than just calming down and going away as mine did. My Girlfriend Amy had great success with the one-two combination of a "vigorous internal examination" by her doctor and then an enema that she gave herself at home later that evening. By about four in the morning, she was pushing the baby out. (Funny, isn't it? I don't mind the thought of someone putting a twelve-inch stainless-steel hook up inside me to break my water, but the thought of an enema makes me feel dizzy.)

Very pregnant women have varying levels of irrationality. I tend to get pretty darned impatient in my desire to move from pregnancy to motherhood, a condition I have always preferred. You may be more restrained, which is an admirable trait in a soon-to-be-mom. You will probably want the baby out as fervently as I did, but your common sense and spiritual tranquillity may allow *you* to accept the unpredictability of the situation. There is something so sweet and sentimental about being awakened in the middle of the night by unmistakable contractions, lovingly nudging your husband awake with the words "Honey, it's time!" and the two of you dashing out in the darkness to your waiting car for your exhilarating ride to the hospital. But, charming as the scenario can be, I always tried to talk my doctor into inducing my labor at a time that was mutually convenient for the baby, the doctor, and me. That guaranteed that the baby would be cooked; my doctor would be fed, rested, and in town; my hair would be clean, my legs would be shaved, and my toenails would be painted. It would also ensure that we made the dash to the hospital in the daytime, with plenty of daylight to help us find our way. Which way is better? My way, of course. Just kidding!

14

What to Take to the Hospital

A Suitcase Full of Useful Things

In addition to yourself, you will need to bring a suitcase to the hospital. Unless your baby comes very early, or you are still having trouble accepting that you are indeed pregnant, you will have a bag packed and ready long before you go into labor. If, however, you need to go to the hospital and your bag isn't packed, JUST GO. Do not worry, because there is nothing you will really need until *after* the baby is born. In the relative calm after the baby is born, you can ask someone to pack a bag for you and bring it to the hospital. If it is your mate who packs your bag, give him a written list specifically itemizing every single article you want. If you just give him general instructions like "Bring me something to wear home from the hospital and some things for a shower," there is a good chance that you will be given a cocktail dress, tennis shoes, a shaver, and shaving cream.

Make it easy on your mate and the hospital staff by bringing only one small (OK, medium) bag. You will probably be moved at least once during your hospital stay, and someone is going to have to move your bag along with you. If you don't have several things with you, you will run less risk of losing something in the move. Don't worry that one reasonable-sized (meaning smaller than a steamer trunk) bag won't hold everything you will need in the hospital, because you really only need something for you and the baby to wear home and a few toiletries. OK, and an iPod, bottled water and snacks for everyone but you, a couple of tabloids, and a box of wet wipes, not to mention the other helpful items listed.

Your Going-Home Outfit

Obviously, I can't know in advance if you are going to have your baby during a heat wave or a blizzard, so I can't pick your outfit for you (much as I would love to). I *can,* however, offer some general suggestions.

1. Wear something that is big, no matter how much you long to wear your old jeans and have your svelte figure back. *You will still be fat,* and you will probably still look pregnant for several days (or weeks) after the baby is born. Maternity clothes are the obvious, though loathsome, choice. Much as this may depress you in the anticipation, it won't really be a big deal when it happens, because at least *someone* will be wearing new clothes in small sizes: the baby. From now on, and for the foreseeable future, no one will be looking at you anyway, at least not when the baby is in the same room.

2. Wear flat shoes. You will be a little groggy and off-balance after giving birth and lying in bed for twelve hours. The last thing you need is to try to safely carry your baby into your house while you are wobbling on a pair of stilettos. Also, you might still be retaining water, and you won't want to be sausaged into anything too tight.

3. Wear a blouse or dress that "breathes" and is absorbent. Checking out of the hospital, putting the baby into a car seat, and heading home all conspire to make you perspire like crazy. And there is always a good chance that the baby will spit up on you at least once before you get home.

Also, if you intend to nurse, make sure that the blouse or dress you choose opens far enough down the front for you to get your breast out without too much trouble. You will have your breasts in and out of your clothes so often in the next few weeks that you will be beyond modesty. You will nurse in the middle of a monster-truck competition and answer the door for the FedEx man (bearing yet another gift for baby) with your breast looking him right in the eye. Most shocking of all, you will soon think nothing of whipping your breast out and nursing your baby in front of your own *father.* Yikes! You probably don't believe me now, but just wait until you have been hiding in your bedroom nursing for an hour while the family reunion has been taking place in the living room without you; you'll come running out like some escapee from *National Geographic*.

4. Look somewhat attractive. You don't need to kill yourself getting all dolled up—as I mentioned, you probably won't be the center of everyone's attention—but keep in mind that your picture will be taken several dozen times between your leaving the hospital bed and entering your home. Go for a little makeup and do your hair, and don't fret one more minute; but do brush your teeth, for the baby's sake. Then hold the baby up in front of your face like a shield and, if all else fails, threaten to destroy the camera of anyone caught taking a close-up of you.

Do Not Bring a Nightgown (Unless You Don't Mind Ruining It)

The Girlfriends' advice is to leave the pretty nightgowns and matching robes at home. Childbirth and its aftermath are bloody, and if you wear your lovely things from home, you will be soaking them in Woolite for the next several weeks. Just wear the hospital gown they give you when you are admitted. Don't worry, you won't be wearing it long, because nowadays new mothers are sent home from the hospital so quickly that they barely have time to do anything more than brush their teeth and take a shower.

Bring Your Own Shampoos, Soaps, and Lotions

After you have given birth, there are no greater delights on earth than taking a shower and brushing your teeth. It will probably have been hours since you have done either, and the effect of feeling clean will be almost as good as losing fifteen pounds. The toiletries that the hospital provides, assuming it provides anything, are industrial and in microscopic containers (à la "the food is lousy and the portions are too small"). Indulge yourself by packing some nice shampoo, shower foam or soap, and lotion. Keep in mind, however, that your new baby has a virgin nose. The little thing could sneeze its head off if you have the whole room smelling like Giorgio. Select mild scents and skip the perfume and cologne altogether. Also, if you are planning to nurse your baby, avoid putting anything on your breasts, be it lotion or powder. After all, how would you feel if someone sprinkled White Shoulders dusting powder on *your* meal?

Leave Your Jewelry at Home

If your wedding band still fits without cutting off circulation in your ring finger, you can wear it to the hospital. Other than that, all jewelry should stay at home, where it won't get lost in the shuffle. You won't even need a watch, because your ever-ready birth coach will have one, and failing that, every maternity room I have ever seen has a huge wall clock like the ones we had in school. Who knows, you may look so naked without your earrings and pendant that your mate might actually be inspired to go out and buy you a little bauble as a reward for your valor in the delivery room!

Bring a Pillow, or Two

We have already discussed the ever-deepening love you will have for your pillows during pregnancy. You sleep with them between your legs, you hug them against your chest, you even take them in the car for your ride to the hospital to deliver. As loving and supportive as they have been up to now, they have never been more worthy of your devotion than when you rest gently on them in your hospital bed. I don't know what hospital standard-issue pillows are made of, but I am tempted to say sawdust or crumbled plaster. Your own pillows will not only help you sleep comfortably (which you most certainly deserve at this point), but they will also help bolster you and the baby at feeding time. Best of all, they smell like home. (Just remember to leave your best white pillowcases at home, for obvious reasons.)

Bring Bedroom Slippers

I know that hospitals are supposed to be all sterile and such, but I have my doubts, especially where the carpets are concerned. When you are just resting in your room, you may find a thick pair of socks sufficient to keep your feet warm and cootie-free, but if you are prodded into strolling around the whole wing to help get your intestines working again, you will want to have some slippers that are flat and comfy and not too ugly. It is definitely best to skip the little mules with the feathers, because your balance may not be too good. Or worse, your legs might actually look good enough to arouse your partner and give him a hankering for sex. YIKES!

For Your Partner

Leave this page open on your partner's pillow or pasted over his toilet:

ATTENTION, DADDIES:

THE GIRLFRIENDS' GUIDE HEARTILY RECOMMENDS THAT YOU SHOW UP WITH A GIFT OF SOME SORT SHORTLY AFTER THE BABY IS BORN. YOU WILL ALMOST NEVER GO WRONG WITH JEWELRY, SINCE IT WILL FIT EVEN BEFORE YOUR WIFE HAS LOST HER BABY FAT. IT INDICATES AN APPRECIATION OF THE VALUE OF THE HEROIC JOB SHE HAS JUST PERFORMED. IF PEOPLE GET GENEROUS REWARDS SIMPLY FOR FINDING LOST DOGS, YOUR WIFE IS NOW ENTITLED TO THE HOPE DIAMOND FOR THE SERVICE SHE HAS JUST RENDERED.

Bring Lots of Socks

My Girlfriends and I recommend that you bring thick socks, and lots of them. You will wear your first pair during labor, a time when lots of women get cold hands and feet, literally and figuratively. Your doctor will probably let you continue wearing your socks during delivery, but you will want to throw them away as soon as your consciousness returns, because they will probably be pretty bloody. The other pairs are for you to wear in bed in the hospital so that when you get up to use the toilet, your little tootsies won't get cold or contaminated. Chances are you will end up tossing a couple of these pairs, too, because you will inevitably sense too late that your diaper has runneth over, and as you streak to the bathroom, there will be blood and watery stuff running down your legs and into your socks. (Don't spend too much time trying to visualize this; just take my word for it and move on.)

Bring Big-Girl Panties

Unlike the socks, you will not need your underwear during labor and delivery, since most doctors agree that they tend to be a hindrance. You will, however, need at least three or four pairs for your hospital stay, no matter how brief. After the baby is born and all the other pregnancy stuff has come out of you, a nurse will put a couple of sanitary pads on you and you will lie in bed on disposable square mats. For the first few hours you might skip underwear, because this is usually when the nurse will bring you ice packs for your swollen peepee. Plus, she will want to look at how you're doing "down there" every few hours.

After the ice-pack period has passed, you will want your own underwear, both for modesty's sake and also to keep those sanitary pads where they belong. For this, we recommend full-cut briefs, even if you were a G-string devotee during your pregnancy. No G-string is going to offer a whit of support for the pads you will need down there to soak up all the liquids that pour out of you for days after birth. And besides, after a vaginal birth and a couple of stitches, you will look upon your favorite thong as a vicious instrument of torture. No, what you need are big, soft granny pants that feel soft and cushy.

Bring Lip Balm

Something about childbirth dries out the lips, even for those of us who did our Lamaze breathing only for the time it took to yell for the anesthesiologist. Certainly you are being dehydrated by losing so much water during the birth, but in addition, you won't be given anything to drink during labor and delivery for fear that it will make you nauseous. If you don't think ahead to bring something for your lips, you will probably end up all chapped and cracked. You can't prevent that from happening to your nipples, but a good lip cream will help your mouth.

Bring a Pen

At first I was going to suggest that you bring paper, too, but then I was reminded by my Girlfriends that between learning to feed your baby, welcoming all your visitors, sleeping, and trying to relax enough to go to the bathroom, you will have no time for composition. If you are deeply committed to your journal, then go ahead and bring it if it makes you feel better, but keep all the thank-you notes and birth announcement envelopes at home.

(My Girlfriend Dorothea suggests, after just giving birth to her second child, that all baby announcement envelopes, or at least labels, should be addressed and stamped during those last boring weeks of pregnancy. Then, when the baby is born, all you have to do is phone in the essential information to the stationer's and later beg your mother or Girlfriends to stuff the envelopes and drop them at the mailbox for you.)

Getting back to the pen, you will be asked to fill out several forms for such things as birth certificates, baby photos, and breakfast menus during your hospital stay. The nurse, after an hour of searching, will generally find a three-inch pencil with no eraser for you to use. Not only will your hand cramp up, but the lead will wear down before you even get to your dinner request. While bringing a pen is by no means essential, you'll find it's the little things that often mean the most.

Bring Something to Eat

My Girlfriend Dona actually had the temerity to tell me that the hospital where she delivered had a *hospitality buffet* set up several hours a day for the maternity patients and their husbands! She suspects that strangers from other wards frequently came in and helped themselves. *Do not expect to find the same setup at your own hospital.* In fact, getting anyone to bring you juice or a snack when it is not a scheduled mealtime is the dictionary example for the word *futile*.

After a task as arduous as delivering a baby, you will be starved. Contributing to this hunger is the fact that your body is getting ready to go into milk production. You will be tempted to accept your husband's sweet offer to dash down to the cafeteria and bring you back something to eat. Keep in mind, however, that you will not see the man again for nearly an hour, because he will tuck into a four-course meal for himself while he is waiting for your tuna sandwich to be wrapped to go. Remember, labor and delivery have taken their toll on him, too.

You will be so grateful to yourself if you have planned ahead and stashed some bottled water, boxed juice, and nonperishable snacks such as granola bars or dried fruit or crackers in your suitcase. Try to avoid the candy bars and cookies at this time. Much as you may love chocolate, your body is sapped and needs more nutritious replenishment. Besides, a lot of babies can't digest the milk of a mother who has been eating Milk Duds all night, so hold off on the junk.

Bring Something to Read

Most hospital rooms have televisions, but if you have time on your hands, you might want to read. Personal experience has shown me that linear thinking is almost totally absent in new mothers, so don't bring anything that requires concentration or memory, because you will have neither. A magazine or two will be quite intellectually challenging, especially if they have complicated things such as the *Cosmo* tests about whether your sex life is as good as it should be, or *Glamour*'s "Do's and Don'ts."

Bring Your Own Sanitary Pads

Things may vary from hospital to hospital, but when I had my kids, I was given the kind of sanitary pads that needed a belt or safety pins to keep them in place. Jeez, I hadn't seen those things since I'd read the book *Growing Up and Liking It.* What a relic! What you need are the maxi-est pads manufactured, with the adhesive strips on the backs. Bring the jumbo box because you will really use them fast, often two at a time, for the first couple of days, *even if you have had a cesarean section.* If you're lucky, the hospital will provide them and you'll never use yours, but better safe than sorry.

Bring a Nursing Bra

If you know that you want to breast-feed your baby, or if you are uncertain but might give it a try, you should bring a nursing bra to the hospital with you. (You will appreciate the support and protection even if you don't intend to nurse, and you should continue wearing your industrial-strength maternity bras, because you will still experience the filling of your breasts.)

Even though babies want to and should nurse right after they are born, they are not getting mother's milk yet. I am sure you have read all about colostrum, the yellowish fluid that the baby sucks from your breasts preceding the manufacturing of milk. You have a wonderful window of opportunity to learn to nurse during this colostrum stage, because the baby isn't starving to death and your breasts aren't too big to maneuver.

The day your milk comes in, all hell breaks loose. I swear, in a couple of hours, my breasts went from soft and full to the size and firmness of a regulation NFL football. I think that the only reason my baby wasn't petrified by these breasts, which were far bigger than his head, was that he was so hungry. That was when I first realized how much I was going to love my nursing bra. I wore one day and night for months because sleeping with breasts that are full of milk can be uncomfortable. Legend has it that Frenchwomen go to bed wearing "sleeping bras" in the belief that breasts deserve to be supported at all times. Now that I have seen how hard a woman's breasts have to work, I think they not only deserve a pretty bra, but a paid vacation for two to the Caribbean.

While we are on the subject of nursing bras, you should also bring nursing breast pads, which are disposable, absorbent circles that catch minor leaks. You slip them into your bra between your nipple and the nursing flap of the bra. They keep your bra clean longer, and the last thing you will be needing when you get home from the hospital is extra laundry.

You might also want to check out a newer contraption called a breast shield. These are cups made out of latex or plastic, and they fit right over your nipples. They not only catch more leakage than the pads, but they keep your bra from chafing against your chewed-on nipples by creating an airspace around them.

Bring a Book on Nursing

Getting a baby to drink from your breasts can be more difficult than learning to use a Cuisinart. I know that it is the most natural act in the world, but I have seen women sobbing over their failure to get the baby to "latch on" properly to the nipple so that the milk comes out. Here is the first news flash for novices: The milk does not just come out a hole at the tip of your nipple, as I had always imagined. It comes out of several little holes all over the nipple, and it only comes out when the baby has it in a viselike grip, with the entire brown part of your breast against the roof of its mouth.

Before you panic, let me assure you that almost every hospital will have someone on staff who can teach you to nurse your baby. Some people are so qualified at it that they are called lactation specialists. This is also where a good book with illustrations can be handy. While your baby is resting and you are still relatively calm, you can study the book. Then when the baby wakes crying and hungry, perhaps you will have a faint idea of what you are supposed to do. Trust me, if you don't seem to have the technique perfected immediately, some nurse is guaranteed to grab your breast in one hand and the baby's head in the other and manipulate them until she gets them both to do what she wants. Your job is to sit there as quietly as possible and watch yourself being manhandled by a total stranger.

Bring a Camera and Film

This is going to be the most incredible experience of your entire existence, and you must commemorate it with lots of pictures. For the rest of your life, you will love sentimentally going over the pictures of the day your baby was born. Nowadays, video cameras are even more popular at birthing parties than still cameras. And we all know people who cherish their videotaped recollections of *every single detail* of the baby's birth. My best advice is that you resist the urge to upload to Utube. My other personal rule is that no camera, still or video, is allowed below my waist, but that's because I don't trust those guys who work in the one-hour photo labs. What if you get famous someday and one of those guys has held on to a few of your negatives? Or worse, what if your six-year-old finds the DVD and mistakes it for his *Lion King* disc?

Remember, labor and delivery almost always last far longer than you will plan for (or can imagine). Therefore, unless you carefully plan ahead, your partner could find himself out of film or with a dead battery just as the baby is coming down the pike. If he is videotaping the event, suggest that he try to save the battery by using the AC plug or, to be on the safe side, by having two or three batteries charged for this occasion.

Many medical people seems to have a touch of the artist, and they are often quite willing to take pictures for you if your husband feels too faint or if he wants to hold his new baby. My son's pediatrician was a terrific photographer. He not only shot pictures during the birth, but he followed the baby into the nursery and then out to meet the grandparents, clicking all the while. Being dressed in doctor's scrubs worked rather like a press pass; he went anywhere and shot anything he wanted without anyone kicking him out.

Bring Your Telephone List

As you can well imagine, several people are going to want to know when the baby is born. In fact, I can think of a few who will not speak to you or have Thanksgiving dinner with you if you fail to call them as soon as the little tyke has been whisked off to the nursery. Chances are, the job of telecommunicating will fall to your husband, since you will be either too tired or too blissed-out to handle something as complicated as a phone. But your partner, too, has just had his universe changed, and he may only remember to call the person he was supposed to meet for breakfast the next morning or might even be unable to recall anyone's phone number.

Your job, in the boring days before your labor begins, is to put together a call list with names and numbers *ranked in order of importance.* For example, first on the list should be *your* parents, since you are the mother here. Then his parents, then grandparents, best friends, and neighbors (if you haven't already called them when you were in labor). Your husband may tire of this chore and not finish the list, but if the calls are ranked, he will at least have hit the most critical ones before falling asleep in the leatherette chair beside your hospital bed or going off in search of food.

One last thing about telephoning people with the news that you two have become parents. If the birth has occurred in the middle of the night, or after 10:00 p.m. or before 8:00 a.m., the only people who will want to hear from you *immediately* will be your parents, siblings, and friends who have kids of their own. Friends who have never personally experienced this miracle will only see this call as an interruption of their slumber and would prefer hearing your glorious news after they have had some coffee.

Bring a Girlfriend

Even though she won't fit into a small overnight bag, do seriously consider bringing a Girlfriend to the hospital with you when you go in to have your baby. Any warm, loving Girlfriend will do, but she would be particularly spectacular if she herself had at some time given birth. As I have been saying since I started this book, having babies is women's work, and having other women around to reassure you, gossip with you, and encourage you is invaluable. If you are really, really lucky, you might have a Girlfriend like Amy, who massaged my feet whenever I had a contraction. I will never forget her calm and tireless presence.

Perhaps you are thinking to yourself that labor and delivery are a private time, for only a husband and wife to share. You worry that you will break the mystical spell by having anyone other than the cocreator of this baby in the room with you. *News flash!* First, your room will be anything but private, even if you have a so-called private room. Before your obstetrician arrives, you will probably have several complete strangers with their hands up inside you. The anesthesiologist will come and go, a nurse or two will be there, and at the end of their shift, they will be replaced by other nurses. Second, labor goes on and on and on, wearing out even the most dedicated partner. About five hours into it, your guy will probably be down the hall chatting with his newfound friends in the waiting room, and you will be watching *Survivor* in between your contractions. Rather than rage at your mate for tiring of this tedium and mentioning for the third time that he is hungry, give the guy a break and have a Girlfriend come and sit with you. If you want to preserve a sacred moment, clear everyone but your partner (who is probably having a doughnut and coffee at this point) out of the room when your doctor tells you it is time to push. Then the two of you can share becoming the three of you.

What to Bring for the Baby

Isn't that a mind-bender—packing things for a person you haven't even yet met? Not that the baby is left naked until you bring it something to wear from home. The hospital will immediately dress him or her in a T-shirt and a diaper, wrap him or her up really snug in a hospital-issue receiving blanket (which I stole and put in my babies' keepsake boxes, for some sentimental reason that I can't exactly recall right now), and sometimes stick a knit stocking cap on that tiny little head to keep him or her toasty warm.

You Must Have a Car Seat!

The only thing that you absolutely, positively, no-negotiating *must* bring to the hospital for taking the baby home is a proper car seat. In fact, hospitals in most states are prohibited by law from letting a baby be discharged until they have been assured that it will be put into a car seat that meets safety regulations, and that the parents know how to use it properly.

A million car seats are on the market, and they range in price from about forty to over a hundred dollars. Some of them are designed to accommodate baby sizes from newborn to toddler through the adjustment of the harness straps and the way the seat is buckled into your seat belts. Really spend some time on this, because a good car seat can be your darling baby's barrier against all the things we are too frightened even to imagine. Ask your Girlfriends, read *Consumer Reports,* and browse through the stores until you find one that you are happy with.

Many of my Girlfriends ended up buying two car seats for their baby. The first one, which was useful for about six months, was the bucket-shaped model intended only for newborns. This shape is appropriate because newborns have no spine or neck control and are comfortable in a sort of curled-up position. You will be astonished at how tiny your new baby will look in a car seat of any kind, and if you buy one of the big ones now, you will feel obliged to sit beside the baby in the backseat and steady its wobbly head with your hands. Remember, the big difference in car seats for newborns and car seats for older babies is this: NEWBORN BABIES' CAR SEATS FACE BACKWARD IN THE CAR. This is because studies have shown that this puts them at less risk for whiplash in a sudden stop.

We Girlfriends all opted for the infant car seats that look like plastic buckets and that latch onto a base that remains buckled into a seat belt of the car. The bucket part where the baby nestles can be released from the base and carried out of the car by a handle, so you don't have to wake the baby up to get it out of the car. This way it doubles as a baby seat for use inside the house. Some of these seats also have sunshades; get one of those if you can, because you will spend the next several months worrying about the sun beating down on your baby's face, both for fear of sunburn and because it makes them so cranky. Consider buying a brand-new car seat (as opposed to borrowing one that your Girlfriend's child has outgrown) because there are often safety improvements with each newer model. In fact, some of the really old models of seven to ten years ago might not even meet current safety requirements.

I want to say one last thing about car seats, then I will get on to the fun stuff: Recent studies have shown that thousands of otherwise intelligent parents are using or installing the car seats incorrectly. READ THE MANUAL! If it says that the seat belt has to be cinched with the "enclosed metal clip," don't throw the metal clip away—use it! If it says that the seat belt has to be inserted through a series of tunnels underneath the car seat, then go through every single one, not just the big one in the middle. Also, don't assume that all car seats work alike. You have to read the manual every time you get a new one. I know it can be irritating to figure out those silly diagrams, but keep reminding yourself that a baby is at stake. So, for once in your life, *read the instructions.* And then, when you are sure you know how the thing works, practice installing it and releasing it several times. Take advantage of your relatively calm state of mind before the baby comes to master this technology.

The Going-Home Outfit, Continued

Picking this outfit is so much fun! The only warnings I have are to pick something that doesn't have too many buttons or need to be pulled over the baby's head, because dressing your newborn for the first time is traumatic (for you, not for the baby). And select clothing that has legs instead of a gown, because the seat belt needs to latch between the baby's legs.

A T-Shirt

Working from the inside out, the first essential is a T-shirt. This shirt should already have been laundered at home (as should all baby clothes, at least for the first three months) with one of the mild baby detergents, like Dreft or Ivory Snow, sold in any grocery store. Some infant T-shirts pull over the baby's head, but for a new mother, the shirts that tie or snap closed on the side like a kimono are far less frightening. For the first few days, pulling anything over your new baby's head will convince you that you are at risk of suffocating it or breaking its neck. Since logic will have little effect on you at this point, I won't bother to reassure you about how resilient your baby is. Instead, I suggest clothing that will allow you to avoid the situation entirely.

In your shopping excursions for the baby's layette, you will encounter T-shirts that pull over the baby's head and snap between its legs. These articles are traditionally called onesies. We Girlfriends think they are great, but not for the brand-new baby. First of all, they involve that neck-breaking suffocation thing. Second, they make it difficult to get to the baby's belly button, to clean it with alcohol until the umbilical stump falls off. And third, the crotch snaps hold the shirt against the belly button, which can't be too comfortable while there is still a stump there.

The Diaper

The next article in the newborn's uniform is a diaper. I have absolutely no opinion whatsoever about whether you should choose cloth or disposable diapers. Living in Southern California, I can't decide whether it is worse to add to the landfills with disposables, or to contribute to the drought and to the chemicals in our water supply by machine-washing cloth ones. All I can really tell you about diapers is to change them regularly, and to fold down the tops to allow that healing belly button to stay dry and free of chafing.

Footsies

You should put something on the baby's feet. For the first couple of days of life, these little creatures have a hard time regulating their body temperature, and their head, hands, and feet need to be kept cozy. You can either dress the baby in pajamas with the feet sewn on, or you can put on the little stretch bootees that are sold in all baby stores and drugstores. Whatever you do, don't plan to put shoes on your newborn. I know these little doll shoes look cute in the store displays, but a real baby's feet are so tiny and rounded that the shoes are irritating to them. Besides, it's nearly impossible to put anything other than a sock on an infant's kicking foot; and even socks won't stay on for long.

The Stylish Part

What you choose to put over the core baby uniform is subject to your own taste (and sense of humor, since baby clothes can be funny). You should, however, know that the vast majority of new babies sleep almost constantly for the first few days. For that reason, it makes sense to dress them in soft pajamas or rompers rather than miniature sailor suits or tiny dresses. It is also helpful to know that the current wisdom has babies sleeping on their sides or backs, so you might choose clothes that button or snap up the front or on the shoulder rather than up the back, where the baby would have to lie on them. And stay away from frills, buttons, and bows for now.

To Cap or not to Cap?

Until a couple of decades ago, it was unheard of to take a child outdoors without a hat or bonnet on. A capless baby was viewed by all the other mothers as a sorely neglected child who was certain to catch a cold. My mother-in-law, who lives in New York, would silently pray to St. Jude when she'd see me take her California grandchildren out bareheaded. I know that if she had been my mother, and not my mother-in-law, she would have threatened to report me to the child welfare offices. But since she didn't want to interfere, she'd surreptitiously shield the baby and put her hands over its head when she thought I was not looking.

She was right; I must admit that babies *do* lose a lot of heat from their heads, so if a chill is in the air, a hat is a good idea. Besides, I love my mother-in-law, so if a cap makes her happy, then why not? (At least when she is around to see.) You don't have to go out and buy tiny caps for your newborn, which can be hard to find small enough or be too expensive, because most hospitals supply a great little knit hat that looks like a long-shoreman's cap. Even more preciously, they come in pink for girls and blue for boys, so they eliminate the tedium of constantly having strangers ask your baby's sex. There is no reason, however, to be overly protective and dress the baby like an Eskimo—unless, of course, your baby *is* an Eskimo.

A Pacifier

Regardless of your preconceived opinions about "binkies," do yourself a favor and buy a couple. (Your hospital may provide them, but don't take it for granted.) You may thank me for this advice when your husband is driving you home from the hospital, you are sitting in the backseat next to the baby, and the baby starts to wail inconsolably. All new parents start to perspire and experience shallow breathing at a time like this. You don't know whether you are supposed to speed up and get home as fast as you can, pull over to the side of the road and take the baby out of the car seat to feed it, or, in desperation, take the baby out of the car seat and hold it in your lap for the rest of the ride.

Whatever you do, **do not drive one inch with the baby out of its car seat.** Not only is it incredibly dangerous, but it is also illegal. An important rule for parents is not to let momentary desperation make you do stupid things. Otherwise you will be facing an entire future of doing stupid things.

Here is what you do: Put a pacifier in its mouth and gently tap its end until the baby calms down enough to suck on it. If you have nightmares about your six-year-old going to school with a pacifier, you can add it to the ever-growing list of things to worry about later.

A Blanket

You will want to wrap the baby in a blanket, even if the weather is mild. This is because being wrapped up nice and tight lets the baby relax and feel protected. When its arms and legs are moving around too freely, the baby feels as if it were falling and its reflex is to jerk to attention. Even in a car seat, you can tuck the blanket around the baby, especially over its hands and feet.

An "Urp Cloth"

My Girlfriend Sondra invented the fetching title *urp cloths* for the diapers or blankets that mothers wear over their shoulders when they are burping their babies. Not only do they serve the obvious function of protecting your clothing from spit-up, but they also protect the baby's face from any irritating fabrics or detergent residues in your clothes. You will also constantly use them to wipe drool or some other baby froth from the little one's face.

These urp cloths get better with laundering, since most cloth diapers start out a little stiff when you buy them. Even better than a diaper, in the Girlfriends' estimation, is the Carter's waffle-weave blanket that is sold in most baby stores. It is such an inexpensive blanket that you can buy several. I used them to wrap the baby in, to clean the baby's nose on, to lay over the car seat, and to put over my shoulder. They became such a familiar part of my wardrobe that I frequently left the house wearing one and not noticing. It was quite the fashion statement, especially if it was soiled.

The Neck Doughnut

A couple of years ago, I noticed a new product in one of the zillions of baby catalogs I receive. It was a small, U-shaped ring made of cotton fabric and stuffed with batting. Its purpose was to support the sleeping infant's head in a car seat, baby swing, or infant carrier. I wasn't sure at first whether this was a brilliant invention or just another useless gimmick to sell to naive mothers-to-be. After using it with two of my children, however, I have decided that it is, indeed, a stroke of genius. An infant's neck is so weak, and its head is so heavy, that a baby sleeping in a car seat looks about to tumble forward at any moment. The neck doughnut gives the heavy head a place to rest and makes a new mother worry a little less about whiplash. As we all know, one less thing to worry about is a gift from God.

Just take care to place it safely away from your baby's face so that it can't ever interfere with breathing.

You may be tempted to bring or buy so much more stuff, but avoid that urge. We moms-to-be know that our babies deserve *everything* under the sun. The truth is, however, that they need little more than us. Amazing, isn't it?

15
Labor Begins (Finally!)

AMONG PREGNANT WOMEN, two concerns about labor are universal: "Will it hurt?" and "How will you know when it is happening?" The answer to the first concern is, yes, it will hurt, but probably not too badly for the first few hours. Of more immediate importance is how to tell if you are about to go into labor—or if you are, indeed, already there.

My Girlfriends and I have amassed as many indications as we could think of that your baby is coming soon, and here they are.

The Nesting Instinct

A couple of days before you go into labor, you may feel an irresistible urge to clean your house or defrost your refrigerator or put all your CDs in alphabetical order or some other such anal task. I am not talking about the normal panicky cleaning fits that some of us fall into when our mother calls and says she is stopping by unexpectedly, or the way you finally get around to putting the broken toilet-paper dispenser back on the wall because your brother and his new wife are coming to stay for the weekend. No, I am talking about the kind of feverish cleaning where you use your husband's toothbrush to scour the pipe that goes from the back of your toilet into the wall. I'm talking about taking off every switch plate in the house and soaking them all in Pine-Sol. This is the time when otherwise rational women truly believe that they cannot sleep one more night in a house where the baseboards have not freshly been painted. This is nature's way of making sure that you will be ready for the new baby, and it is called nesting.

A week after her due date, my Girlfriend Mindy was discovered by her mother tottering at the top of a six-foot ladder, feverishly sponging down the shelves at the top of her closets. To indicate how out of character this was, I have to tell you that Mindy's "baby" is now seven years old (nineteen as of this second edition), and that those shelves have never seen a sponge since. Mindy's alarmed mother tried speaking soothingly to her, much as one would talk to a person standing on a skyscraper ledge threatening to jump. "Are you sure that's such a good idea, dear?" she asked. "Why don't you come on down and let me do that for you?" But Mindy was powerless to stop, and completely unable to see how bizarrely she was behaving.

My Girlfriend Sondra started cooking as she neared her delivery date. She calmly and rationally explained that she just wanted to have a few meals frozen, so that her husband could microwave them when she was in the hospital and when she first got home. It made sense, until I saw Sondra's car in the grocery store parking lot at 7:00 a.m., waiting for it to open. She made so many casseroles that she filled her own freezer and soon spread out to her Girlfriend's across the street. When she tired of casseroles, she decided it was imperative to provide some variety for her lucky husband, so she taught herself the intricacies of Chinese cooking in the predawn hours before the grocery store opened. Then she moved on to barbecuing everything she could get her hands on, even if it meant standing outside in the rain holding an umbrella over the gas grill. Let me cut to the chase: Sondra went into labor, went to the hospital, gave birth, and came home before her husband had time to eat one single lasagna, and she celebrated the birth of her daughter by making Belgian waffles for her parents and in-laws only six hours after the baby was born. (OK, so maybe Sondra's not such a good example.)

One morning at dawn near the end of her pregnancy, my Girlfriend Shirley's husband woke to find her side of the bed empty. Convinced that she was in labor or giving birth in some other room in the house, he leapt naked from the bed to find her. She didn't answer his calls, and he couldn't find her anywhere in the house, even though her car was still in the garage. Then he looked down the steep hill that many people in Los Angeles refer to as their "backyard." There was Shirley, pushing and pulling a wheelbarrow filled with fertilizer up and down the hill. Her baby was going to come home to a house with grass, by God, and she had been working toward that end for hours before the sun came up. No mere gardener could be trusted with fertilizing *her* baby's lawn; no, it was *mother's* work.

Windowsills and shutters became my obsession during one pregnancy. I was determined to eliminate all dust from all rooms, and I bought several contraptions to brush it up, wipe it off, or filter it out of the air completely. One night, I awoke feeling as if I had been electrocuted—I had the sudden realization that all the dust I had brushed off the sills and shutters must have landed in the carpet. My husband had to physically restrain me from ripping up all the carpet in the house. I had to be satisfied with having it professionally cleaned, TWICE.

My Girlfriend Jillian, who expresses her nesting instinct in ways more artistic than antiseptic (and who has a cleaning lady to help with the more mundane scrubbing matters), started frantically putting all her loose photos in albums and desperately trying to bring up-to-date the baby books of the two children she already had when she was waiting to deliver her third. (By the way, this baby-book thing can be a real burden, especially after the first baby. Pretty soon the book becomes little more than a storage folder for all the clippings and doctor's reports and report cards that you can jam in it, everything out of order and unattached. Take it from me: All mothers have deep-seated guilt about unfinished baby books. And if they don't, they have way too much time on their hands—or, more likely, no baby books!)

Anyway, getting back to Jillian, there she was on the floor, surrounded by photographs and albums, with a pregnancy the size of a world globe on her lap, trying to make some organization out of this memory chaos. Her understanding (or fearful) husband passed by several times, but dared not suggest that maybe a nap would be more beneficial. No, Jillian had a mission and would glue-gun anyone who thwarted her. Wouldn't you know, she slipped the very last photo into the very last album, then heard a little pop. Her water had broken, right on cue.

General Pissed-Offedness

Another indication that you are rounding the homestretch may be a persistent and increased crankiness. I know, I know—pregnant women are accused of being emotionally unpredictable frequently during the entire nine (ten) months of their pregnancies. But there are a lot of good reasons why you should be particularly cranky at this point: (1) You are not sleeping much or well; (2) you are bored with being a biology experiment; and (3) you feel oppressively aware that there is no backing out of this delivery thing now, and you are beginning to suspect that the baby is much easier to deal with while it is inside you than it will be when it is on the outside.

But my Girlfriends and I think there is something even more unique about these last few weeks of crankiness; something that, to the experienced eye, indicates that *this woman is about to erupt.* Think of her as a volcano; she is a big old mountain of a thing, but from the outside you can't tell if she is dormant or filled with seething lava. Only a thin trickle of steam indicates that she is about to blow.

I remember seeing my Girlfriend Maria at a children's birthday party right before the birth of her son. When I went up to say hello, she looked as if she couldn't quite place me, even though we had been friends for ten years. To the casual observer she must have looked calm to the point of being nearly unconscious, but to the other mothers in the crowd, she was clearly going to have that baby within hours. Her intuition was telling her that she was about to undergo the greatest challenge and transformation of her life, and she seemed to be hunkering down in preparation.

As they face the biggest task of their lives, many women begin a subtle kind of withdrawal from their everyday life. They develop what I call the Stranger in a Strange Land Syndrome, where they go through the motions of their usual business, but feel distanced from and uninvolved in it. Things that they would normally find amusing become trivial or irritating. They are sick and tired of being pregnant. They want to get the ordeal of birth going so that they can stop dreading it, once and for all. This is a good time for friends and family, especially husbands, to stay out of the pregnant woman's way as much as possible, and to answer yes to anything she asks, because any confrontation now is bound to be messy. She has entered the "zone."

My Girlfriend Julee, who is a manicurist, was the brightest, cheeriest pregnant person you have ever seen. Every week, I would try to pry one single complaint out of her, and every week I was disappointed. To her, nausea was a minor inconvenience, heartburn was something to be endured with good humor, and she still didn't know what hemorrhoids were. Then came her last three weeks. Overnight, the old Julee had been snatched away, and in her place was a woman who spent the day with her head down, looking at the hand in front of her. She filed and painted those nails with such fervor that you would think she believed each stroke was bringing her that much closer to the end of her pregnancy. She had begun the long march, and she was prepared to deck anyone who stood between her and her destination. All of the gossip and chatter that flew around her in the manicure salon just sailed right by her. She didn't seem to hear any of it, and if she did, it must have seemed completely meaningless and trivial given what she was facing.

The Baby Drops

That certainly sounds dangerous, doesn't it? But the change is subtle and often barely noticeable. At the end of your pregnancy, you might notice the baby is sitting lower in your stomach than before. This is because it's starting to lock into the birth position and is being held in place by your uterus. This generally only happens with your first baby, because in subsequent pregnancies your weakened stomach muscles "drop" the baby the minute it gets heavy. Dropping is also referred to by some as "lightening" (for reasons that I will never understand, because absolutely nothing is getting "lighter" at this point).

Like so many things in pregnancy, dropping is a good-news/bad-news proposition. The good news is that you will find it easier to take a deep breath and fill out your traumatized lungs. The bad news is that for your lungs to be liberated, your stomach and bladder have to be sacrificed. From now on, you will get full long before you finish a serving of food. You will also constantly feel as if you were about to wet your pants, but when you sit down to relieve yourself, only a teaspoon or two will come out.

Diarrhea

Some of my Girlfriends have told me that their tummy felt crampy all day before they went into labor, and that their stools were all loose and watery. We concur that it can be hard to tell the difference between diarrhea cramps and early labor contractions. In fact, as we Girlfriends think back on it, we believe that they were probably the same thing. For this reason, it is wise to pay particular attention to a funky tummy in your third trimester. Just as you feel the need to clean everything before your baby is born, your intestines also seem to have a nesting instinct. Often, shortly before or during the early stages of labor, you may find your bowels wanting to clean out anything you may have eaten in the last twenty-four hours. If it happens to you, be grateful, because this evacuation means you are off and running, and because there will be less poopoo on the delivery table when you push. Until recently, it was traditional hospital procedure to give all delivering women enemas. Since then, the prevailing wisdom has been that a little poop never killed anyone.

Passing the Mucus Plug

The mucus plug is exactly what it sounds like: a kind of bloody, snotty thing that corks up your cervix so that no nasty germs get through to your uterus while the baby is in there growing. The thinning of the cervix and the beginning of its dilation can leave the plug no longer big enough to fill the hole, and out it comes! I will never forget my Girlfriend Lorraine screaming for me from the bathroom when she was very very pregnant. "Look in there," she cried, pointing into the toilet and staring into the bowl bug-eyed. "What is *that*?" I, who had not yet had children myself and had never seen anything so disgusting floating in a bowl, just stood there dumbly and held tight to her arm, because I was certain at least one of us would faint.

There are two important things to know about passing your mucus plug. First, labor will soon begin, but not necessarily immediately. Many Girlfriends have passed their plugs and not gone into labor for a couple more days. And second, this is only a good thing. It doesn't hurt, and since it usually happens while you are sitting on the toilet, it doesn't even make a mess. Oh, yes, one last thing: Not everyone passes her mucus plug before active labor and delivery. I have never seen my mucus plugs, and believe me, I have peered into many a toilet bowl hoping to find one.

Your Water Breaks

Everyone has heard this expression with regard to pregnancy, but few of us know what to expect or recognize it when it happens to us. Of course, *water* doesn't really break, but the *membrane* that has been filled with water for your little baby to float around in for the last forty weeks does. This is the result of a uterine contraction or the baby's head pushing against it and popping it. Sometimes it pops like a water balloon, with a gush of water soaking you, your clothes, and wherever you have been lying or standing. Other times the bag just springs a leak and you feel a constant trickle of water between your legs. Either way, the universal sensation is "I'm peeing, and I can't stop!"

My Girlfriend Jillian says that when it happened to her, she rushed to the toilet. She peed so much that she reached behind her and flushed the toilet halfway through, because she really worried that she would fill the bowl and it would overflow onto the bathroom floor. And this is a mother of *four*, so you know that this birthing business is just full of surprises. What contributes to the sensation that the water supply is unending is that it is, indeed, unending. Your body replenishes the water (placental fluid) at an astonishing rate so that the baby doesn't get dry and pruney, or more important, so that infection doesn't set in, so you can really dribble away for hours.

Since about half of all expectant mothers will have their water break at home, it is a good idea to prepare for its happening to you. One particularly good idea is to put a mattress protector or a plastic sheet on your bed. (Your water tends to break in bed and really gush because the baby is relaxing on your spine or side when you sleep.) Then, when you stand up, the flow will stop or slow down a lot because the baby's head will go back down on your cervix and act like a drain plug. The other suggestion I would make is to always wear a sanitary napkin during your last few weeks. One napkin, even a super-duper maxi, definitely won't be enough to soak up all the water, but it will give you running time to get out of the checkout line of the grocery store and into a bathroom.

Two important things you should know about your water breaking are:

1. It does not hurt at all!
2. You must call your doctor and get ready to go to the hospital, because this event will only end with a baby coming out. You can go for a few days without your plug, but if you are near or past your due date, your doctor will probably not want you to walk around with your water draining out for more than a few hours.

Dilation and Effacement

By the time you have delivered your baby, you will toss around these two words with great casualness, but for now, let me explain what they mean. *Dilation,* which we Girlfriends agree is the more important of the two, refers to the stretching open of the cervix, the short tunnel that connects your uterus to your vagina. *Effacement* describes the shortening of that tunnel in preparation for birth. By the time you are ready to push, the tunnel that is the cervix is so short that it's not so much a tunnel anymore as it is a sort of membrane between the uterus and the vagina. And in dilation, this membrane is stretched wide enough for a baby's head to come out. Dilation is measured on a scale of one to ten. If you are one or two centimeters open or dilated, that baby isn't going anywhere. By the time your cervix is open ten centimeters wide, which theoretically means the doctor can stick all ten of his or her fingertips inside the opening, it's bombs away!

Unless you are a contortionist, you cannot determine for yourself if you are dilating or effacing. These are things your doctor will report to you during your last few office visits. For first-time mothers, there is tremendous satisfaction in calling your friends and family to announce that your doctor has just told you that you are two centimeters dilated and 25 percent effaced. With that kind of news, labor is certain to be right around the corner, right? Well, not necessarily. Millions of pregnant women are on the streets right this very minute, walking around two and three centimeters dilated, and their babies may still not come for another week or two (or even three). Sorry!

Other very pregnant women forlornly leave their doctor's office after being told that their cervix is closed up tight as a clam, only to go into active labor that same night. So my advice is this: If you are effacing and dilating, go ahead and get excited, because the least it can do is relieve your boredom. And if you are not changing at all in there, do not worry one little bit, because it doesn't mean a thing. By my fourth pregnancy, I walked around for weeks so dilated that my vagina made little squeaking noises with every step, and it felt as if the baby's head were between my thighs. But did the baby come early? Not by one second!

Contractions

The confusing thing about contractions is that they come in all forms and intensities. I would estimate that 99 percent of us go into labor having absolutely no idea what to expect. And when it begins, we all wonder, "Is this *really* it?" The Girlfriends' rule of thumb is this: If you think you might be in labor, stay calm. Rarely does a first baby slip out ten minutes after the first contraction, so there will probably be no need to call 911 at this point. It is important, however, that you don't be a Labor Martyr, either. If you feel unusual in any way, pick up the phone and call your doctor, even if you just saw him or her two hours ago. Believe me when I tell you that doctors *expect* you to rely on them to tell you if you are in labor or not. Call them; it makes them feel needed.

The Myth of False Labor

This is probably a good time to talk about false labor. The most reassuring thing I can tell you about false labor is that it is a myth. That's right, hogwash. It's just one more thing to make you feel that you are ignorant and out of control when you are pregnant. *All contractions are contractions, and all contractions are preparation for birth.* Some just occur closer to the time of birth than others. Therefore, you are not a moron if you feel contractions, go to the hospital, and then get sent home. It happens all the time. It simply means that these contractions you are feeling are not *noticeably* dilating and effacing your cervix, and you might have a few more hours or days before things start opening up in there.

My Girlfriend Sondra had me drive her to the doctor when her second baby was due. We really flew down the freeway, because she was having contractions, and since she had already had one baby, she knew what labor felt like. Half an hour later, we were sent home empty-handed; no open sesame. A week later she felt contractions again, but this time they were stronger and more regular, so she skipped the doctor's office and met him directly at the hospital. Wouldn't you know, still no open sesame. But by this time Sondra had had enough of this torture, and she refused to leave the hospital. She informed her doctor, with a hint of hysteria in her voice, that she would not go home until she had a new baby to take with her.

In fact, your uterus has been contracting ever since your egg got fertilized, but you probably didn't really start noticing it until the middle or end of your pregnancy. The contractions that do not noticeably open up your cervix are called Braxton Hicks contractions. They are designed by God to get you in the mood for labor. Toward the end of your pregnancy, your uterus will frequently contract, with increasing intensity. Sometimes your belly gets so hard and rigid that you could bounce a dime off it. Most pregnancy books say that Braxton Hicks contractions do not hurt, and compared to productive contractions, this may be true, but my Girlfriends who had a lot of them say they were by no means painless. While they may not feel like a knife stabbing you in the tummy, they can be serious enough to take your breath away and make you feel the need to sit down or lean against something. And early labor can feel exactly the same way, so you can see why it's so easy to get confused.

Some women feel mild cramping contractions for a full day or two before their contractions get compelling enough for them to go to the hospital. My Girlfriends Janis and Tracy both felt kind of punk, as though they were getting the flu or their period (remember those?), when they were in the early stages of labor. They called their doctors to check in, then casually kept an eye on the clock to see if their moments of crampiness had any regularity or pattern. In the meantime, they called their families and hung around the house. My Girlfriend Patti had these mild contractions at first, too, but she had no intention of waiting all day in her house for something to happen. She and her husband went to a matinee movie, then to the hospital.

My Girlfriend Amy never had time to buy a box of popcorn, let alone see an entire movie, because her labor always came out of the clear blue sky and with the intensity of a thunderstorm. With the first contraction, she knew it was time to go to the hospital, and by the time she got there, she was already feeling the urge to push. Her description of trying to take off her cowboy boots in a tiny hospital bathroom while in hard labor is really funny (cowboy boots are problematic even under the best of circumstances). A quick, efficient labor can be good and bad. It is good if you dread a long-drawn-out, tiring labor, but it is bad if you have your heart set on an epidural, because there won't really be time for one.

If you are feeling the flulike, period-like symptoms (and your baby is due, of course), and you would like to try to move things along a bit, walking could be a good idea. If you don't feel like walking, however, sleep is equally valuable, and a little nap might be the perfect thing. Some women will have irregular and relatively manageable contractions for more than a day. The pains are not strong enough to make them rush to the hospital, but they are too strong for them to get any sleep. If this happens to you for more than twenty-four hours, your doctor might prescribe a sedative or sleep medication so that you can get some rest before the final rounds of labor begin.

You might want to eat something light, because once you get to the hospital, it's ice chips and cotton swabs that taste like lemon until you get that baby out. Chances are, you're so excited and nervous that food is the last thing on your mind, but a little soup or a milk shake couldn't hurt.

Scheduled C-Section

One other persuasive indication that your baby is coming soon is a scheduled C-section. With a scheduled C-section, you and your doctor have agreed to a time at which you will enter the hospital in a fairly calm and leisurely fashion, and he or she will extract your baby through a small slit at the top of your pubic hair. There are a lot of reasons to schedule a cesarean section, including medical conditions such as placenta previa (don't ask), breech babies, or twins or triplets. Other women elect to have a cesarean because they want to maintain the vaginal tone of a teenager, and their doctors find medical explanations that will suit their insurance companies. And then there are those women who temperamentally just cannot take the uncertainty that waiting for labor to begin entails. If they are lucky, their doctors, too, will help them contour their insurance policies to cover this planned delivery.

Of course, I cannot have a clear conscience unless I remind you that it is actually better for the baby to be born vaginally, for many reasons. The squeezing helps force the fluid out of their lungs, you will need less anesthesia (if you consider this a *good* thing), and your recovery will be quicker. Still, C-sections are safe for mother and child, and the recovery time is surprisingly short.

Yes, I read the papers, and I am aware of the outrage in some quarters about the number of unnecessary C-sections that are performed in the United States. Am I resentful or indignant? Not particularly. The temptation will be extraordinary for you to feel that you would rather have your fingernails pulled out by their roots than succumb to a C-section. You will be convinced that the big emotional payoff of pregnancy lies in the physical challenge of laboring and delivering the baby vaginally. Gingerly, I suggest that you not set these expectations for yourself. A significant number of women who have their hearts set on vaginal births will end up having C-sections, and there is absolutely no reason for this to be a source of disappointment.

As someone who has had babies both ways, I must admit that I don't really have a preference for one over the other. Having a healthy baby was all

I really wanted, and I didn't care how I got it. However, by the fourth child, I was begging my doctor for a C-section in the fear that if I had any more big noggins come through my vagina, my husband would be able to yodel and hear his echo down there. My doctor then gave me the disappointing news that it is the *first* vaginal birth that does most of the stretching, so I grudgingly agreed to let yet another one come down the pike (and made him promise to stitch me up very, very well afterward).

So now That You Are in Labor, What Should You Do?

All of the popular books on pregnancy will tell you not to rush off to the hospital too early because they will hook you up to an IV and not give you anything to eat or drink. It is also suggested in these books that, once you get to the hospital, you will be forced to lie down. This is considered a bad thing, because lying down is one of the least productive postures for a woman in labor.

I would just like to say that I was *never* asked to lie down when I was in labor, at least not until I went for the epidural, and then it was a tremendous relief to lie down. In fact, after the baby was born, a nurse was at my bedside within hours telling me I had to get up and walk around. But I digress. . . .

If you and your doctor agree that you are fine and comfortable laboring at home for the first few hours, that is wonderful. I, however, love maternity wards. I love all the new mothers, the pictures of babies on the walls, the nursery full of babies, the abundance of trained medical professionals. I cannot think of a place where I would rather be in labor, no matter how many hours lie ahead of me. You have a choice: You can walk around your own house to help your labor along, or you can walk around the hospital. At least at the hospital, you won't feel compelled to make all the beds and unload the dishwasher while you walk. And you won't have to rush to get there later.

TOP 10

Ways to
Deliver Babies

10. In a Scientology Silent Birthing Room with Tom Cruise as the Birth Coach.

9. When You're NOT in a Car or on an Airplane or at a Sporting Event That Serves Beer on Tap.

8. In a Hospital Room Where Your Cell Phone Works.

7. On an Empty Stomach (Sure, You'll Get Hungry, but Since the Proper Pushing Technique Is like Pooping, It Could Cut Down on the Mess; Even Though No One Really Cares Except You).

6. With Your Lipstick and a Small Mirror in Your Partner's Pocket.

5. With Clean Hair, No Roots, and a Fresh Pedicure.

4. With Someone at Your House, Cleaning and Cooking for Your Return.

3. With Dr. McDreamy as Your Obstetrician.

2. Sipping on an Epidural Cocktail and Watching *Oprah*.

1. Via FedEx.

16

Going to the Hospital

ALL RIGHT, GIRLFRIEND—here we go! You and your doctor have reason to believe that your baby is on its way, and it is time to go to the hospital (or whatever other professional birthing center filled with competent and caring medical people you have selected). I swear, this time is so filled with excitement, fear, and anticipation that no astronaut getting ready to enter a space capsule has ever felt more anxious. It isn't liftoff yet, but from now on, everything leads to this ultimate conclusion. This is what you have been building up to and preparing for nine (ten) months, but you still don't really know what to expect, even if you've already had kids.

A general suggestion for women about to have babies is to try to get a shower in before liftoff, because it will be quite a while before the opportunity will arise again. If you are not laboring so hard that you risk giving birth on your shower tiles, hop in for a quick shampoo and underarm shave before leaving for the hospital. The two rules in this area are:

1. Do not take a shower if you are alone in the house, because you may decide midsuds that it wasn't such a good idea after all and you might need someone to help you out.
2. Do not take a bath if you have any reason to think that your water has broken, because you may introduce bacteria into your uterus. Besides, if you think getting out of the *shower* while experiencing contractions is a challenge, wait until you try hoisting yourself out of a tub.

The Drive

I know that you have never even considered this, but it will make me feel better if I just say it: DO NOT TRY TO DRIVE YOURSELF TO THE

HOSPITAL. Even if you think that the contractions are bearable and that you are perfectly fine to drive, don't get behind the wheel, because conditions in labor have been known to change quickly. Also, women in labor are rather like people who have been drinking: They think they are acting normally and are in control, but they should *not* be allowed behind the steering wheel of a car under any circumstances. If your mate isn't home, call a Girlfriend, a neighbor, a cab, or 911. One revelation that almost all of my Girlfriends had was that the car ride to the hospital is a bigger deal than they had imagined it would be. In their meticulous planning and anticipating, they had pictured what they would do at home and what they would do at the hospital, but the car ride in between had been an inconsequential detail. Then, when they were actually in labor and in the car, they realized that this ride might be a challenge in itself. It can be as uncomfortable as a ride in a wagon with square wooden wheels.

First of all, sitting upright with a seat belt around you is not the most comfortable position in which to labor. If your front passenger seat reclines, put it back as far as it will go. If it doesn't, ride in the backseat, where you can sprawl. Do try to wear your seat belt, even if you are reclining or leaning in the back. Your driver will be particularly nervous and prone to slamming on the brakes unexpectedly, so being strapped to your seat will help you cope. Besides, you haven't come through the last nine (ten) months in pure and perfect health only to get injured in the car ride to deliver the baby.

Like the princess with the pea under her mattress, you will feel every pothole and piece of gravel in the road during this ride. You will also be feeling a tad irritable, so you will probably curse the Department of Public Works the whole way (when you are not silently cursing your darling husband for turning so sharply, stopping so abruptly, and getting you pregnant in the first place). One good way to counter this is to bring your bed pillows from home, as many as you can carry. (You will not only love their familiar comfort during the car ride, but you will continue to appreciate them in your hospital bed, where they traditionally top the bed with some wafer-shaped thing that they have slipped into a pillowcase.) Put one pillow under your head and one between your legs, and try to rest on your side in the car. (Once again, the left side is the politically correct one, but at a time like this, embrace any side that works for you.)

Try turning on the radio. Its familiar music or mundane chatter might be reassuring and might distract you from whatever discomfort you may be feeling. It will also help relieve you of the obligation of keeping up a conversation with your husband, who will be as nervous as you are. An old doctors' rule of thumb is that if you are experiencing a "productive" contraction, you will be unable to speak during it or at most only be able to make strained, high-pitched noises. As soon as the contraction passes, you will return to your garrulous, or complaining, self. So if you are in active labor during the car ride, your conversation will be punctuated by contractions. If the radio is irritating you, ask your husband to turn it off, even if it's your husband's favorite song. Be creative in your endeavors to be comfortable. Try silence, try asking your husband to tell you a story or a joke, try singing "A Hundred Bottles of Beer on the Wall." Heck, you could even try out those Lamaze skills and see if you think they are going to get you through this ordeal. (Why waste valuable time at the hospital when you could be getting your epidural?)

Bring a bottle of water (room temperature is best, because you will be less inclined to get stomach cramps from it) to sip along the way. Once you are checked into the hospital, you won't be given another taste of that glorious liquid until the baby is on its way to the nursery to be measured and weighed. (Even then, it will be a challenge to flag down a nurse or orderly to get you something to drink, because the doctor and nurses seem to magically disappear along with the baby.) Don't drink too much or too fast, however, because you might get nauseous, and the only thing worse than having contractions in a moving car is vomiting at the same time.

Checking into the Hospital

Please don't hold me to the details because every hospital has its own routines and policies, but what follows is a general description of what happens once you get to the hospital.

Under ideal circumstances, you have preregistered and handled all your paperwork and insurance stuff weeks ago. Also ideally, labor is progressing at a manageable pace, and you have had time to call your doctor and he has told the hospital you are coming. Under these conditions, you will go to whichever admissions desk handles maternity patients, a bit of information you will have learned beforehand. Within seconds you will find yourself seated in a wheelchair, whether you want one or not. Don't start arguing or making a scene about the wheelchair, because it's required by the hospital's insurance policy. Besides, if you start out complaining and arguing, you may piss off someone upon whose mercy you will later have to rely. Shut up, sit back, and enjoy the ride.

If you have not been preadmitted to the hospital, you may have to check in via the emergency room. Don't worry—they move visibly pregnant women right to the head of the line here, no matter how many broken legs are ahead of you. After a quick check-in, you might be taken to an area called triage. This is usually a larger room with several nurses and several beds (divided by curtains, if you are lucky). In triage, you are examined and put on a monitor to see if you are having productive contractions. If you are, then your doctor is called and you are sent to a labor room. If you are not, you will be told to get dressed and go home. If this happens to you, please do not be too discouraged, and don't be in the least bit embarrassed. I can describe triage to you because I have been there a couple of times myself and have been sent home, even though I had already given birth to two children and you might have thought I would know better.

My husband hates triage, and he wants me to warn you about it. Every time we have been there, some woman has been in the bed next to me moaning and crying in labor, basically scaring him to death. If that happens to you, just mind your own business and repeat to yourself, "I am just fine. The woman next to me is no indication of how my own labor will go." Trust me—these words are true, and there is no sense in letting someone else's fear contaminate you. You *will* be just fine. And by the way, so will she.

The trend in consumer-pleasing hospitals is to make the labor and delivery rooms more homelike and less surgical. Often, uncomplicated deliveries take place in the same room where you have labored. Do not take this new development for granted; in the not-too-distant past, right when you least wanted to move (like when your contractions were coming one on top of the last), you were taken from a labor room to a bright and sterile surgical room to deliver, with stirrups and everything. I had my last two babies in rooms with televisions, telephones, a stereo, and even lights that could be dimmed. It was divine.

Once you are admitted either to triage or to your labor room, you will be given a big plastic bag and directed to a bathroom to change into a hospital gown. The plastic bag is for you to put your own clothes and shoes in. Yes, you must take off everything, including bras, panties, and watches. You may, however, keep your socks on, and you will be grateful for this small comfort.

At this time you will meet someone who will become an important figure in your life: your labor and delivery nurse. This person—more than your doctor, more than your husband, and certainly more than any book on pregnancy—will help get you through this ordeal. Trust her advice; she has been through this birthing business hundreds of times and knows what she is talking about. If the angels are smiling on you, she will be a Girlfriend by the time this ordeal is over. Mine, Estelle, is still my friend and our kids are in school together sixteen years after our first delivery.

On the slim chance that you discover immediately that you can't stand the nurse who has been assigned to you, beg your husband to see if you can trade her in for another model. Don't make it about *her* being mean or insensitive or having bad breath. Now is the time for you to be humble: Say that *you* are hard to get along with, and you are so sorry to be so irrational, but you simply can't help yourself. The Girlfriends believe that you should do your best to avoid offending anyone who might be called on later to save your life. Trust us—later on, when you are about to push, the chances are good that you will offend or insult several people. Just make sure that your nurse is someone you can rely on and trust, you know, like the Ultimate Girlfriend.

Soon after you have changed into hospital garb, you will have a fetal monitor strapped around your belly like a belt. This is fun, because it communicates your contractions to a machine beside your bed and shows the baby's heartbeat. Please be warned that changing positions, either yours or the baby's, can interfere with the monitor's ability to detect the heartbeat. *This does not mean that anything is wrong with the baby.* It just means that the belt has to be adjusted.

You will probably have an IV needle placed in the back of your hand or forearm and connected to a bottle of saline solution. The rationale is that the saline keeps you from becoming dehydrated, and that if you need any other medications quickly, the doctors already have a tap in place. Some of my Girlfriends made a real fuss over the IV, as if only a sadist would add to a laboring woman's discomfort by sticking her with a big needle. Others, such as myself, found labor and impending birth to be so overwhelming that I barely noticed it.

Hurry Up and Wait

After the initial excitement of settling in and hooking up, you will probably not have much to do. Especially with first babies, labor tends to go on
for hours, punctuated by a doctor or your new best friend (your nurse) occasionally reaching inside you to report how dilated you are, or are not. If
you're not too uncomfortable, try to rest because pushing a baby out is a
surprisingly athletic feat and you will need your strength.

Now is a good time for your Girlfriends to drop by or to phone them,
because you might be a little bored (at least when you are not having a
contraction). Nearly every one of my Girlfriends was shocked by how
long and how hard the contractions have to be to get your cervix dilated
enough for a baby to come out. It is so common for a Girlfriend to labor
for six hours and endure contractions that make her see stars, then be told
she is only four centimeters dilated. It feels as if you were running a race
where they keep moving back the finish line, which can really rock a
woman's ability to cope.

You may also be stricken by the fear that you are not physically strong
or athletic enough to give birth after all. Keep in mind what I told you earlier: This is not a fitness test, and you will manage to get that baby out,
even if someone has to sit on your stomach to help you push.

You might think to yourself, "I can take this pain if someone will promise me it will all be over in two hours." That's the problem—no one will
know how much longer your labor will last, and that can be dishearten-
ing. Try not to focus on the labor at this point, but on the prize at the end
of the race: a precious baby placed in your trembling arms. Remember, to
paraphrase *Annie,* the sun and the baby will come out tomorrow, at the
latest.

How Much Does Labor Hurt?

Early labor is like the worst case of menstrual cramps you can imagine,
but with more total-body involvement. A good contraction is so overwhelming that you will be unable to do anything else but contract. Not
only will you not be able to talk, but you will not be that crazy about listening, either. Several of my laboring Girlfriends have yelled "Shut up" to
their husbands and other visitors because their conversation irritated them
during a contraction.

As labor progresses, it can take on a variety of personalities. You may have heard of someone's traumatic "back labor," for example, when the baby pressed against the mother's spine. Other women describe contractions that came so close together, they didn't have time to prepare for the next one. Generally, however, when women talk about the pain of labor, they are referring as much to the marathon of pain as its intensity. One hour of hitting yourself with a hammer may hurt a lot, but fifteen hours of it will certainly make you delirious. We all agree that the hardest part is not having any idea how long you will have to bear up. The fear that the pain might continue indefinitely is what usually brings down even the strongest of us. We would give anything if only someone could guarantee that there were only seventy minutes left (like on the StairMaster).

The other thing that can break down a laboring woman's control is nausea. I bet no one ever told you about that, right? Well, Girlfriends, it is extremely common for laboring women to feel sick and throw up, especially as they near that final part of labor called transition. Think of this as one more way that nature has of cleaning you out in preparation for birth. Do not think of it as abnormal or an imposition on anyone (except you, that is). Simply tell the nurse or nearest person that you are sick, and you will be stunned at how quickly a basin or a towel appears under your chin. Think of vomiting as a respite of sorts, an interruption of our regular programming that will leave you feeling lighter and better.

Pushing

I have a Girlfriend, a professional woman of intellect and experience, who actually told me she didn't realize that you have to push to get a baby out. She thought that the contractions would be hard enough to move the baby down the birth canal, without any extra work on her part. Boy, was she surprised. Pushing is real physical work, and it can take anywhere from a few minutes to several hours. Once you are dilated and fully effaced, a nurse will stand at your head and a doctor will stand in the catcher's position, and they will coach you through this athletic feat.

On each contraction, you will grab your knees or thighs with your hands in an effort to fold up tight and make as little room for the baby in your lap as possible. On the assumption that this won't be enough to give him the hint, you will also push down with every muscle between your chest and your knees. The sensation that will immediately come to mind is that of making a bowel movement.

Congratulations—you are doing it right! You can really be sure of your technique if your face is squeezed so tight that you feel as if you were giving yourself crow's-feet all the way to the back of your scalp. Don't worry for one second if you feel as if the baby were coming out of the wrong hole; at a time like this, any hole will do. (Besides, he or she probably has a better sense of direction than you think.)

If you don't take any pain relief, either because you don't want it or because your doctor has determined that the baby is coming too fast for it to be of much use, the most terrifying moment of your life comes when you are told it is time to push. As much as nature is already making you feel like bearing down, you are way too smart to think that moving that baby out of your vagina isn't going to hurt. Imagine a burning sensation involving your entire crotch area, combined with stretching that makes you think your hips will break—or better yet, don't!

Now catch your breath, because I am going to tell you the one and only way to make this pain subside: PUSH RIGHT THROUGH THE PAIN AS HARD AS YOU CAN. That's right—do the opposite of what your mind is telling you to do, which is to lie still and whimper. This will take a tremendous amount of courage on your part, but I promise that it will help. Either it will activate a pain-numbing mechanism that nature provides when the baby's head pushes through the cervix, or it will simply get the whole ordeal over with sooner rather than later. One thing I can tell you for certain: Lying there and repeating "I changed my mind, I changed my mind—I don't want a baby!" will provide absolutely no relief. Now is finally the time when your husband can really join in and help. He can push you into a sitting position with each contraction to help you bear down, or he can help you and the nurse hold your legs in the up-and-ready position (you'll resemble a frog, by the way). Then again, helping you may interfere with his camera duties, so you'll have to delegate the various responsibilities.

The Epidural

The most common method of pain relief for a laboring woman is the epidural, a combination of drugs released into the fluid surrounding your spinal cord through a needle in your lower back. As you are reading this description, you are probably so alarmed that you are convinced you would rather go through labor sober than to have anybody sticking needles into your spine. After a few good hours of hard labor, however, you would probably welcome an epidural even if it was administered through your eyeballs.

An anesthesiologist must administer an epidural. The good part about this is that no amateurs will be puncturing your spine and crippling you for life. The bad part is that not all hospitals have anesthesiologists on duty twenty-four hours a day, so there may not be one around when you want one. My Girlfriend Chris decided at the last minute that she didn't want to do an unmedicated delivery of her third child. She had gone the frontier-woman route with her previous two babies, and she had nothing left to prove to anyone. She asked her doctor to call an anesthesiologist to give her an epidural. Unfortunately, he was at home asleep, and by the time he got to the hospital, Chris was holding Baby #3 in her exhausted arms. The lesson here is if there is even a remote chance that you will want an epidural, tell your doctor several times during your pregnancy and remind him or her when you call announcing that you are in labor. Then say it again, over and over, to anyone in scrubs from the minute you arrive in the hospital until you feel that tap in your back.

When given an epidural, you will either roll over on your side or sit on the side of your bed with a nurse bracing you for support. The doctor will then have you curl up in a ball as best you can under the circumstances; this separates your spine so that they can get to the magic spot. Chances are you will have a contraction sometime during the procedure, but they will be patient and wait until you can lie completely still. Then you will be given a shot of novocaine in your back. Moments later, the doctor will put a thin shunt into your back and tape it in place. You may be surprised to learn that an epidural is like an IV, in that it remains in place in your back during the rest of labor and delivery. That way the anesthesiologist can monitor your pain level and administer more or less of the drug accordingly. You can lie on the shunt and roll around, and you won't feel or disturb it.

You will probably feel the sensation of an electrical shock running through your legs when the epidural is first activated. Don't let this frighten you. It is momentary and completely normal and will not, in retrospect, even register on your pain-o-meter. After the zap has passed, the relief is almost immediate. You will be infinitely grateful and astonished when you see another contraction registering on the graph paper from the monitor beside your bed while you feel nothing more than pressure. This is generally when pregnant women get their personality back. They become nice and loving to their husbands, and chatty with their nurses and Girlfriends. Even better, many of them are able to take a nap.

Wonderful as an epidural can be, it has a couple of little drawbacks. The most immediate one is that it tends to slow down productive labor. The other is that you may be so numb from the waist down that you cannot push hard enough to get the baby out. For this second reason, the anesthesiologist might turn down the epidural when it is time to push, so that you can be of some assistance at this critical juncture. Or you can try what my Girlfriend Janis did. She swore on the life of her husband that she would find a way to push without feeling if they would just promise not to turn down her epidural. The doctor agreed to give it a try, and Janis *willed* that little girl out, through sheer terror.

Pitocin

You might be dilating at a centimeter an hour, get an epidural, and then fail to dilate any more for quite some time. This is when the drug pitocin might be administered. Pitocin is dripped into your system through the IV in your hand, so no new puncturing is required. The drug is also used to induce labor when the doctor and mother mutually decide that the baby has overstayed its welcome. It usually brings on contractions that are hard and constant—so hard and constant that women who have bravely been laboring without pain medication scream for the epidural if they have been given pitocin. Any notions of "hee-hee" Lamaze breathing through these contractions will usually result in hyperventilation and tremendous frustration, but, hey, you can take my word for it or decide for yourself when the occasion presents itself.

An Alternate Route

All the pitocin and laboring in the world just may not result in your cervix's opening up enough for the baby to come out. You are probably a dishrag at this point, and even your baby may be showing signs of fatigue. Then comes the suggestion that you have dreaded for nine (ten) months: "Maybe we should consider a C-section." This suggestion is almost universally met with great disappointment and alarm, usually manifested in a sobbing fit. Suddenly your dreams of childbirth are shattered. Your hopes of meeting the physical challenge and emerging victorious are shot. This disappointment and feeling of failure are almost always more upsetting to women than the prospect of having their stomach cut open with a knife. I have Girlfriends who, years after their C-sections, still feel robbed of one of life's great experiences, who still think that if they had been allowed to labor "just a little longer," the baby would have been born vaginally.

Please don't start restricting yourself now with expectations and rules about what denotes a "successful" delivery and what denotes a "failure." A delivery that results in a healthy mother and baby is a gift from God, no matter how that delivery was achieved. Period. Childbirth is not like a visit to a spa: It is not designed for your personal enjoyment and fulfill-ment. It is not an opportunity to demonstrate your abilities or fitness. It is designed to perpetuate the species, and nothing more.

If you and the doctor determine that you are going to have a C-section, your epidural will be turned up. If you don't have an epidural in place, you will immediately be given one, or, if time is critical, you will be put to sleep with general anesthesia or given a spinal block. I have had a C-section with an epidural, and the sensation I remember most was all the jostling about. I felt no pain, but I did feel as if I were being moved around, inside and out. And I was surprised at how long it took to get the baby out. I am sure they can do it faster if they have to, but a leisurely C-section consists of methodical incisions through each individual layer between the outside world and your baby, not one deep cut right to the baby. Once the baby is delivered and its umbilical cord is clamped off, you will probably be given some long-lasting painkiller such as morphine. The rest is euphoria, at least until the morphine wears off.

Birth

Since I am a "mature" mother (read "older"), I have had genetic tests that revealed, among other things, the sex of my baby. Some women choose not to have their doctors tell them this information because they want to be surprised at birth. I still find everything about giving birth surprising or shocking, and I don't need to add one more thing. Besides, I like to start decorating the nursery as early as possible, so I have always known whether I was having a boy or a girl. You might not know, however, and here is your big moment. With that last exhausted push comes the announcement "It's a boy!" or "It's a girl!" Make sure that you hear the definitive statement from a medical person, because fathers are notorious for seeing the umbilical cord and mistaking it for a penis. Only trust those people who have their anatomy knowledge certified by a medical degree.

I have no words to adequately describe the feeling of seeing your baby the moment it emerges from your body. Even if you are exhausted and disoriented from labor and medication, looking at the creature who has been living inside you all this time will be the closest thing to seeing God that life can provide, without the help of a burning bush or a parting sea. In all your imaginings, this is probably where your movie ended, with your baby being put into your arms, you and your husband gazing lovingly into each other's eyes, the music swelling, and the credits starting to roll. Sorry to be the one to tell you, but that is not exactly how it goes in real life. . . .

If you have had a vaginal birth, the baby might be placed on your belly for warmth while the doctor clamps the umbilical cord and someone (perhaps your baby's daddy) cuts it. Then you still have some pushing to do, because the placenta has to come out, too. If you have had a C-section, they take the placenta out for you, so lie back and relax. After you have pushed out the placenta (and a lot of other bloody, gucky stuff that can look alarming but is perfectly normal), the doctor will reach inside you to see if anything is left that might cause infection. This part is not fun, and it usually comes as a surprise to a new mother, who wants to be left in peace after what she has just endured. Breathe deeply for this part or ask the doctor to turn up the epidural.

Then comes the stitching. Chances are, if you had a vaginal birth and it is your first, your doctor performed an episiotomy before the baby emerged. That means he or she made a slit in your stretching skin to make more room for the baby to come out. The justification for this is that if the cut weren't made, the baby would tear you anyway, and it's theoretically easier to stitch up a clean slit than a ragged tear. My experience was that I ended up with episiotomies *and* tears, so I had more stitches than Frankenstein's monster. The stitching part usually doesn't hurt, but it does take a while. So while your husband and the nurse are having fun with your baby, you are lying with your knees wide-open and your precious parts being sewn back together.

Love at First Sight?

You may take one look at your new baby and sob with the depth of love and devotion you immediately feel. Or, you may take a look to make sure it is whole and healthy, then secretly hope that some professionally trained person takes it away somewhere. This does not mean that you will not love your baby as much as the next mother does, or that you have the character of a slug, so take it easy on yourself. Birth is traumatic, even under the best of circumstances, and you may need a while to allow your emotions to catch up with your new identity. Think of it this way: Even your dearest friend may have taken a while to work her way into your heart, and she didn't give you stretch marks—so why should you feel obliged to fall in love with this little stranger the minute you lay eyes on it? Just know that it will happen, and you will grow to feel a love so fervent that your insides hurt and you can't take a deep breath without its catching.

Now What?

Your doctor and nurse will leave once they finish putting you back together as best they can. Your baby will be taken to the nursery to be given an injection of vitamin K, weighed and measured, foot- and hand-printed, and having other such bureaucratic stuff done to it. It will also be evaluated for its alertness, reflexes, strength, and, in our family, sense of humor. The result of this evaluation is called your baby's Apgar score. I don't want to say much more about it, because tests and evaluations give me performance anxiety.

You will be moved from the birthing room to a regular hospital room. During your stay, your time will be spent putting ice packs on your swollen privates, resting as much as possible, learning to nurse and change diapers, and receiving visitors. You won't realize it for quite some time, but this enchanted period ends much too soon. In fact, in about three months you will long to check back into the hospital, where your meals (albeit tasteless) are prepared for you, your sheets are cleaned every day, and your baby is taken away by capable professionals whenever you get tired. The Girlfriends advise that you stay in the hospital as long as your insurance allows you to. Even if it's just one more day, that is twenty-four hours of postponing the inevitable: a lifetime of work and responsibility.

17

Postpartum Dementia

The Small Potatoes

It really is shocking, but the hospital or birthing center is eventually going to turn over a helpless, fragile, and needful human being to your care. So, counting you and your husband, that makes three of you. With less training than you got when you learned to insert your diaphragm, you are expected to go home and raise this baby to adulthood. (If you are not frightened at this prospect, then you certainly don't have a vivid imagination.)

As alone as you may feel at this moment, most of your fears have been experienced by Girlfriends since the beginning of the ability of the human animal to be neurotic. And if their words aren't enough to get you started worrying, all you have to do is watch daytime television, because every talk show and news broadcast will be about some child-related disaster. What follows is a list of some of the most common paranoias about mothering.

"I'll Break Its Neck!"

We have heard so many times that newborns have no ability to support their own head that we live in fear of their little noggin jerking out of our careful grasp, snapping off their neck, and rolling onto the floor. So far, in all my research, I have never heard of a mother accidentally injuring her baby by letting go of its head. It is true, however, that you should hold the baby with two hands, because they frequently jerk their heads unexpectedly and can fall backward out of your grip if you aren't paying attention.

The most anxious moments (truly terrifying in the beginning) are when you are dressing or bathing the baby, because a newborn's head feels at least as heavy as the rest of its body parts combined.

The companion worry to "I'll break its neck!" is "I'll squish its head!" The entire top of a newborn's head is soft because the bones of the skull haven't joined together over the top. You will have no problem being gentle with this area, but every one of your Girlfriends' little children or your own older kids are guaranteed to pat on it hard with their grimy mitts—or more likely, with a wooden block. Don't wait for the Girlfriends to notice and stop their darlings; just grab away the offending hand and sweetly say, "No, no," through your clenched teeth. Better still, hold your baby out of reach, especially when that danger is another child.

"As Soon as We Stop Watching the Baby, It Will Stop Breathing!"

Just wait until you see how many times you'll stand beside your sleeping baby and stare at it as if its lungs were only working through the sheer force of your will and concentration. New mothers are terrified of something dreadful happening to their babies while they aren't on watch. If the mother happens to have enjoyed a particularly restful snooze of three straight hours, she will fly to the baby in morbid dread that it must have died, to allow her to sleep so long. Heaven forbid that the baby is quietly sleeping, because the frantic mother will have to pinch it awake to hear it cry before she can be satisfied that all is well.

"I Will Forget I Have a Baby and Leave It Somewhere!"

I have had several vivid dreams in which I put the baby in his car seat and sat it on the hood of my car while I dug in the diaper bag for my keys, and then, after finding the keys, I jumped into the car and sped off, leaving the baby sitting on top of the car. One of my Girlfriends used to fret that she would take her baby shopping with her and then accidentally leave it in a dressing room, not realizing her mistake until she got home. There are several variations on this theme of failing to care for your baby in the most fundamental ways. My Girlfriend Chrissie used to have nightmares that she would drop her baby over a hotel balcony. It would happen in slow motion and she'd be powerless to stop the sequence, even though she knew how it would turn out. Let me hasten to reassure you that Chrissie's kids are nearly grown now, and obviously the products of truly great parenting, so the dreams were not the sign of a sick mind, but simply the sign of a mother who was afraid of how much she loved and wanted to protect her kids. OK, and maybe just a pinch of postpartum depression.

"I'll Sleep Through a Feeding and the Baby Will Starve to Death!"

A startling (at least to me) number of new mothers rely so completely on the feeding schedule that their pediatricians suggest to them that they feel obligated to wake a sleeping baby to make sure it doesn't miss a feeding, as if it will perish without those precious four ounces. Babies don't really perilously exist from feeding to feeding; they are meant to be slightly more durable than that. The only time I can think of to wake a sleeping baby to feed it is when you are breast-feeding and your breasts are threatening to explode if someone doesn't suck the milk out quickly.

Remember, the goal is for your baby to learn to sleep all through the night without needing to eat. Relax and be grateful if the baby has skipped the traditional 11:00 p.m. feeding; he or she will eat enough at the next feeding to make up for it. Wake it during the day if you must, but not at night. Babies usually get one decent stretch, so it is better for everyone concerned if that stretch comes at night, after all the good (or at least watchable) television shows are over.

"What If the Baby Doesn't Like Me?"

A lot of Girlfriends, particularly those who had a mother's helper or grandma to help them with the baby for the first few weeks, said that they worried that their baby liked the caretaker better than them. They said that the babies cried more or were restless when they held them, but calm and sleepy when someone else held them.

I can't offer any guarantees for fifteen years from now, but at this age your baby loves you with every ounce of its existence, because you are what stands between it and a difficult world. It may not love you for your wit and charitable deeds, but it will love you as part of itself. There is nothing you have to do to earn this love; it's far more fundamental than that. Your baby has to love you—it's the rules. He might just be reflecting your own nervousness when he fusses. Or, more commonly, he is simply expressing his excitement at the meal that awaits him, since you smell like a milk wagon to him. If your baby loves other people in addition to you, don't be selfish; there's plenty to go around.

"What If I Don't Like the Baby?"

You will always love your baby, but you may not always *like* it much. A mother who has been walking the baby up and down the hall for five hours without being able to get it to sleep may be close to wanting to sell the little one. If our friends or our spouses were as demanding and selfish and oblivious to our personal happiness, we would drop them like hot potatoes. You haven't *seen* neediness until you have had a baby; this is the Grand Canyon of need. And what do they give you in return? A crooked smile now and then, perhaps a dirty diaper. When you feel a cloud of resentment sinking down around you, ask some benevolent soul, such as your mother or husband or Girlfriend (don't you just love your Girlfriends?), to take the baby somewhere where you can't hear it or see it for an hour or two. The respite will work wonders.

"Why Is My Life Such a Mess?"

Even the most finicky and organized of us lose all control of our environment when a new baby comes home to live with us. You will wonder, as you step over piles of laundry on the living room floor, how one tiny baby can require so much time and work. Forget writing thank-you notes and returning phone calls; you are lucky if you get a shower in, and a miracle worker if you put on clothes that actually match and are clean. Generally, you look crummy, the baby needs something, and you and your partner haven't eaten anything but Lean Cuisine in three weeks. Then your mother-in-law calls to say that Aunt Grace has asked her five times whether you got the *Pat the Bunny* book she sent you, since she *still* hasn't heard from you.

This is the real postpartum depression—not that wimpy, little tearfest the books say you might experience in the hospital after the baby is born. All this, combined with about two solid months of sleep deprivation and sore nipples, can really get a Girlfriend bummed out and possibly give her a nasty cold. I wish I could give you the secret cure to this condition, but there isn't one. The best advice we can give you is to accept your limitations, and accept your friends' and family's offers of assistance. Sure, they may drive you crazy or be completely unable to find their way around your kitchen, but let them try, because they are still more capable than you are. Just know that we have all suffered what you are suffering, and we sympathize deeply. This, too, shall pass (just much more slowly than seems humane).

"I Hate Nursing!"

It is politically correct these days to breast-feed our infants. The justifications are numerous and reverently listed in every other book on pregnancy. The Girlfriends' position on breast-feeding is this: Try it. If you like it, keep doing it. If you don't like it, you have our permission to quit. The world is filled with women who rank failure to nurse right up there with child abuse, and they love telling you about how they nursed their own children until they were ready to start school. These stories, even to Girlfriends who nursed, are boring and judgmental and should not be allowed to make you feel guilty about your decision. Is breast-feeding better than bottle-feeding? Sure, I guess so. But then, so is baking your own bread, making spaghetti sauce from fresh tomatoes, and never drinking coffee.

The reality is, nursing can be painful at first. It also requires a mother to handle all the feedings by herself, unless she becomes proficient at pumping. As far as I am concerned, a nursing woman is still a little bit pregnant; her body is still working for someone else's benefit. Some Girlfriends have also mentioned that their husbands have a hard time feeling sexual about them while there is a baby sucking on their favorite playthings. No judgments here, just the facts.

So, if all these things are true, why do women ever choose to nurse? Well, it is home cooking at its finest for a little baby. It is also simple, once you have mastered the technique, to open up your shirt, feed the baby, and button back up. No dishes to wash, no ingredients to buy, and it's a lot cheaper than formula. In the middle of the night (*middle* meaning any time of the day or night after you have had at least an hour and a half of sleep), when your hungry baby cries, one of the last things you will want to do is warm up a bottle of formula. It is much easier to just whip out the breast and doze while the baby suckles to its heart's content. Another great medical benefit for the mother is that nursing helps shrink your uterus back to its normal pear size after it has been stretched to the size of a duffel bag.

Now here is one thing you might not know about nursing, but we Girlfriends swear it is true. After the sore nipples are healed and you know what you are doing, nursing feels really, really good. I am talking about good the way sex feels good. When you nurse, a hormone is released in you that has a sedative effect. That slightly drunken feeling, combined with the gentle contraction of your uterus (like after an orgasm), can lead to one deeply satisfied mother. That's why so many nursing women have a goofy smile on their face.

Another less glamorous chemical is released that will make you thirstier than if you had eaten ashes. When nursing, or before you lie down to get some sleep, make sure that you have a large (about the size of a bucket) glass of water at your side. My girlfriend Dona used to take a huge glass of ice to bed so by the next nursing period the water wouldn't be lukewarm.

For me, the best thing about nursing was that it forced me to prioritize my life properly to make room for the new baby. Nursing forced me to neglect the meaningless busyness of my life and pay attention to the baby and me. One of our greatest mistakes as mothers these days is to rush our recovery from pregnancy and childbirth. If it took us nine months to build up to this condition, we should give ourselves at least that long to get out of it. We are rushing things by having a baby and trying to be back to our former life just six weeks later.

"What If I Have to Go to the Bathroom?"

This basic function of the human body will provide your first physical crisis since the baby was born, either vaginally or by C-section. The thought of moving your bowels and passing something of substance down that particular passage will make you shudder. This reminds me of a compelling reason to have a vaginal birth, if you have the choice: You can't leave the hospital after a C-section until you have earned your release by showing your nurse a bowel movement of your making. With a vaginal birth, they will release you with little more than a promise to poop sometime in the near future, in the privacy of your own home.

You will probably still be sore down there, and certainly not eager to stretch out any of the healing tissues. But poop you must! Some doctors will recommend that you take a stool softener daily, beginning the day your baby is born, to mitigate the discomfort. What they should really prescribe is a tranquilizer, because the anticipation is almost worse than the deed. A couple of days after the baby is born, you will get that unmistakable feeling that your body is getting over its trauma and is ready to "move" again. If you are a chicken, as I am, you will try to ignore this sensation until you are on the verge of exploding, and then you will tearfully go to the bathroom like Anne Boleyn going to the chopping block. You will be certain that a bowel movement is going to rip your episiotomy stitches, and that it will not help your hemorrhoids one little bit. But just as during delivery, there comes a time when you have no option but to push, no matter how faint and sweaty you feel. It is over quickly, and you will survive without any tearing, even if you do bleed a little. Does it hurt? Yup, but I promise, it won't hurt like this again, at least not until you have your next baby. Your hemorrhoids may not be too happy, but that's what those little, round, medicated pads were invented for.

"What If My Guy Wants to Have Sex with Me?"

Let's make a pact among all the Girlfriends of the world right now: Even if your doctor tells you at your six-week checkup that it is all right to start having sex again, **you must not tell your partner.** All Girlfriends must agree to tell them that they may absolutely not have intercourse for three months.

For heaven's sake, the doctor's exam itself will nearly have you hanging from the ceiling. Sexual pleasure at this point is an oxymoron. Why, you may ask, would a healthy, sexy woman not want to make love after the baby is born? Well, here are a few reasons that come quickly to mind.

1. Fear of Pain
Two hemorrhoids and about five thousand episiotomy stitches can make your labia and vagina feel like ground beef. There is also a certain amount of bruising and swelling in your perineum, the area between your vagina and your anus.

2. You May Still Be Bleeding
For the longest time after the baby is born, you will experience the never-ending period. At first it is copious and red and rather clotty (pardon me,

but accuracy dictates a certain amount of vulgarity here). With time, it changes to brownish and then yellowish. Depending on your sexual tastes, this may be off-putting to you or your husband.

3. Dry as a Bone

A new mother's vagina is so dry that it needs a humidifier. Your hormones will suspend the production of any lubrication whatsoever, especially if you are nursing. It seems obvious to me that the Grand Plan of Nature intended that mothers of little babies not get pregnant again until the first baby was able to survive in the world, so it made us unsexual. Feel free to try this biological explanation on your horny husband; maybe you will have more success with it than some of my other Girlfriends.

4. Not in the Mood

Becoming a mother is so physically and emotionally overwhelming that it is quite tempting in the beginning to make an entire universe out of just you and your baby. After a day of having a little person suck on you, burp on you, and otherwise help itself to your body parts, the last thing you may want at the end of the day is to have your amorous spouse do the same thing. You just don't feel like shaving your legs and putting on sexy lingerie; you want to lie in bed all by yourself, in sweats, watching sitcoms and with absolutely no one touching you. Contributing to the lack of interest in sex is the small matter of what you look like for the first couple of months after the baby is born. It will probably be several more weeks before your stomach stops drooping when you roll onto your side and your nipples stop scabbing (if you are nursing), and you may be a bit frustrated that you still don't look like *you.* You know for certain that *you* wouldn't want to have sex with someone as out of shape as you, and you can't imagine why your husband would, either.

5. You Are So Tired You Could Cry

Most of my Girlfriends agree that this is the single greatest impediment to resuming a normal sex life after the baby is born. If you have time for sex, then you have time for a nap, and the nap will sound far more enticing for the first few months. You will be tired because you are recovering from the ordeal of childbirth, you may be tired because your body is working hard to keep up the milk supply, and mostly you will be tired because YOU ARE NOT SLEEPING! The fatigue that comes from existing on catnaps and never even having time to dream anymore can make you demented.

6. Fear of Drowning Your Husband

Let me be the first to share with you one of Mother Nature's practical jokes: Sexual stimulation and orgasm can trigger a nursing mother's let-down reflex. This means that, right when things are getting good during sex, you might start squirting milk all over the two of you. Think of the sensation as something like having sex in a car wash. Perhaps you should try keeping your bra on (with extra nursing pads in place) while you ease your way back into the saddle again; yet another reason to postpone this act.

There, now that *The Girlfriends' Guide* has managed to reinforce your dread of having intercourse ever again, let us help you out of this mess. I promise you, you *will* want to have sex again sometime (and the sooner the better, as far as most husbands are concerned). I have put together a few of my Girlfriends' suggestions to break the ice.

1. Get Away from the Baby for at Least an Hour Before You Even Think of Having Sex

You must really break out of the "mommy cocoon" and get reacquainted with your partner. It may seem impossible for both of you, but do try not to talk about the baby during this preparatory stage. First of all, you will miss the chance to really catch up with each other, and second, thinking of the baby may cause your milk to start leaking out.

Now is the time to express to your husband how fragile you are still feeling, and how much you would appreciate it if he would take it nice and easy, in spite of his eagerness. Begging, bribes, and threats are completely acceptable at a time like this.

2. Have a Glass of Wine

I would have suggested this anyway, but now there is even a recent medical study indicating that wine is an aphrodisiac for women. I think most of my Girlfriends have known this all along, but even if it weren't the case, wine would be good, because it helps you forget what you were worried about in the first place. It may still hurt a little when you have sex, but if you are tipsy, you won't care as much.

3. Moisten Things Up Down There

It is not enough just to inebriate, you must also lubricate for your first sexual reunion. Several gels are available over the counter for this purpose, so go out and stock up in advance. Otherwise, you will find yourself rummaging through your medicine cabinet and making do with something icky such as petroleum jelly or baby oil—or worse, using something from the kitchen pantry. A variation on this lubrication idea is to begin the reunion with a massage. I am sure you could use one at this point, and no husband is going to miss an opportunity like this. He is probably so eager that he would agree to do an oil change on your car first, if you made it a condition of having sex. Don't just use regular old hand lotion; buy massage oils from a specialty store. My Girlfriend Sondra, sly thing, gave me *edible* massage oils. Think of them as dessert and let your imagination run wild.

4. Don't Forget the Birth Control

Let me join in the chorus of people who should be telling you, YOU CAN GET PREGNANT WHILE YOU ARE NURSING, AND YOU CAN GET PREGNANT EVEN IF YOU HAVEN'T HAD A PERIOD YET. Consider using a condom (especially if you are nursing and can't take the Pill), because the lubrication of the condom helps ease things along.

I don't think I have a single Girlfriend who can honestly say that she had an orgasm during this first postpartum encounter. Well, maybe my Girlfriend Melanie did, but she also gave her husband oral sex in the hospital only a few hours after having a C-section, so she doesn't count. In fact, it's a mystery to me why I still like her so much. Anyway, the goal at this time is intimacy and affection, not sexual fireworks. I know it may be hard to imagine ever reclaiming your former sexual passion, but you will, I promise.

The Large Potato

I have chosen to call the first few months after a mother delivers her baby (or babies) Postpartum Dementia because until Brooke Shields and Marie Osmond started talking about postpartum depression (PPD), any free-falling felt by a new mother was usually dismissed as "just a case of the baby blues." What a crock of denial that was. I was among the first to stand up and say that my feelings of isolation, fatigue, disconnectedness, and dread were more than the blues or a momentary funk. (I mention this to show my own desperation, not to give myself props.) I was really in an altered mental state and had no way of seeing it at the time. My husband didn't see it clearly, either, and I lied to my obstetrician and pediatrician during my visits. "How is it all going?" they'd ask. "Great, fabulous! It's the happiest time of our lives," I'd say with all the sincerity of a droid.

In the twelve years since this book first came out, doctors, shrinks, and mommies have become aware that the hormonal tsunami of birth and recovery is frequently strong enough to sink a new mom's ship. We also know that this sense of drowning is code red for us to get to our doctors and get help. If we don't realize yet that we've capsized, it's up to our mates, Girlfriends, mothers, or any other aware and loving people to drag us in without our full compliance. If necessary, those around us should call our OB and give her a heads-up, because she can find a pretense to beckon us in and surreptitiously get to the heart of the matter. The motivating sign of my Girlfriend Lili's possible PPD was that this fashionista wore denim overalls every day—to Christmas parties, to fancy luncheons—EVERYWHERE.

I think of PPD as a problem that lies in wait for most of us. Some of us are absolutely going to succumb no matter how satisfied and fulfilled and connected we felt during pregnancy. Others of us, like me, and perhaps Brooke, had pregnancies that were vaguely unnatural and had the air of science fiction attached. IVF, hormones, drugs, bed rest, C-sections and the like all made us feel out of touch and out of control of our pregnancies from the beginning. Then, lack of sleep, a deep-seated feeling of overwhelmedness, and guilt at our lack of gratitude conspired to let us fall prey to PPD. And, once we've fallen, it can be nearly impossible to get up again without help.

Now we all know the signs:

1. Feeling resentful or distant from our baby
2. Worrying that we may harm the baby or ourselves, even without intending to
3. Hopelessness
4. Wanting to sleep all the time or having chronic insomnia and jitters
5. Not eating or bathing or dressing every day

6. And anything else that makes us unable to rejoin the human race or to find joy in anything once we've given birth.

Even my dogs' vet knows the signs that suggest that counseling and/or medication may be called for. BTW, people always say the politically correct "counseling and/or medication," including myself just now, but if truth be told, it's an *and,* not an *or,* situation. Antidepressants, whether short- or long-term, are nearly always suggested, if not outright prescribed and jammed down your throat. This is a biological, physiological, and psychological issue, not an issue of character, personal strength, or ability to love fully. It's a mental health issue, a temporary one—to be dealt with on a medical and an emotional level. Ninety-nine times out of a hundred, mothers with PPD never do a thing to harm or inconvenience their baby, but the wear and tear on the mommies can be immeasurable.

It's way past time to consider PPD, whether mild or extreme, a matter of choice or personal control. I'd even go so far as to suggest that almost all of us get it, at least in a mild form, and that to say that we're happy and we know it, clap our hands, is like rowing up Denial. Just be ready and surrender, Dorothy. You will still be eligible for the Mother of the Year Award, I promise.

18

"The Old Gray Mare, She Ain't What She Used to Be"

THE TRUTH IS SIMPLE: Having a baby fundamentally changes your body (and your mind, but that is a book unto itself). You can (and will) lose every pound you gained, you can do sit-ups until you have the control of a belly dancer, and you can Kegel your insides until they are strong enough to crack walnuts. But you will never be exactly the same as you were before. I hear some women out there disagreeing with me, and they will soon be sending me pictures of themselves in string bikinis to make their point. Save the postage! I'm not saying that you won't look as *good* as you did before. In fact, you may look *better*, but you will not look the *same*.

Girlfriends have told me stories about having curly hair until they had a baby, then watching as their hair went straight as a board. Others have said their skin changed from dry to oily, or vice versa. Lots of them complain that their hipbones are never again as narrow as before the baby was born. My personal gripe is my belly button, which is no longer a perfectly round innie. But more about the things we cannot change later. First, let's talk about the things we can change now.

Losing the Weight

You all know that the only way to lose weight is to stop eating so much and to start exercising like a fanatic. You are just wasting your valuable time trying to measure fat grams and live on SnackWell's. So eat well, but in small portions, and exercise every day.

What *The Girlfriends' Guide* would like to add to the body of wisdom is this:

1. It will take longer than you think. Just to be safe, start thinking in terms of nine Months Up, nine Months Down. The weight will come off, but since all pregnancy weight is not baby weight, it will come off more slowly than you might wish. The good news about giving birth is that most of your big belly goes away immediately. The bad news is that once it's gone, you will notice all the other places where you got fat, such as your arms, behind, thighs, and face.

2. You will have forgotten what you used to look like. I swear that this is the reason why so many women just stay about seven pounds heavier than they were before they got pregnant; they simply don't *remember* how slender they actually were, and they will settle for a reasonable facsimile of their former self. The only foolproof test to see if you have truly lost every pound is to put on your oldest pair of jeans and wear them for a few hours. If they don't give you a wedgie or a muffin top, then you have reclaimed your old figure.

3. You will not get your old figure back until you stop nursing. This flies right in the face of everything nursing advocates will tell you, but the Girlfriends and I stand by our statement. Yes, it is true that hundreds of calories are burned every day that you nurse, more than you would burn on any treadmill or stair-climber. So in the beginning of your weight loss experience, nursing will be your friend.

When you are down to the last five or ten pounds, however, your old friend turns on you. nature absolutely refuses to let go of the fat deposits in your upper arms, your thighs, and, of course, your breasts until you stop nursing. That way there is little danger of the mother running out of the fuel she needs to keep the milk factory operating.

4. Even when you have lost the pounds, you will have to wait for nature to take her own sweet time about tightening your flabby skin back up and pulling your hips back together again. You know that cereal commercial where they ask you if you can "pinch an inch"? No matter how thin you get, you will be able to get a good *handful* around your middle for several months. Or, if you have had four kids as I have, you can carry that extra skin with you to the grave.

5. Do not get pregnant again until you have lost all the weight from the first baby. There is no capital punishment connected to this law, so don't get panicky if you fail to obey it, but the basic rule is, any extra weight you are carrying when you get pregnant again is *yours,* and you are no longer entitled to call it baby fat. Of course, we think you can safely use that term for a good nine months without inaccuracy.

The Legacy of Pregnancy

Now it is time to talk about the physical changes that result from pregnancy that you cannot change, at least not without the help of a good surgeon.

1. Bigger Feet

This isn't a universal experience, but it has happened to enough of my Girlfriends to make it worth mentioning to you. I don't know if carrying the extra weight of pregnancy flattens your feet or stretches the ligaments in some way, but most of my Girlfriends have gone up at least half a shoe size after having a baby. Don't worry, this doesn't seem to happen with each successive pregnancy, so you won't have to change your entire shoe wardrobe every time you have another baby. I am embarrassed to tell you this for fear of sounding even more frivolous than I actually am, but it may really be advisable to weed out your too tight shoes after the baby is born and *throw them all away,* because your feet will not shrink. From now on, on your new, larger foot, comfort should prevail over vanity.

2. Smaller Breasts

Actually, it is probably more accurate to say "thinner" breasts, because the skin remains the same size, but a lot of the fat that used to fill it out is gone, gone, gone. There is a debate about whether this condition is made worse by nursing, but my observation is that it is the pregnancy more than the nursing that takes the toll.

If it is any consolation, when you get pregnant again, you will have another nine (ten) months of great tits, but the end of the story remains the same. I have only one word of comfort: Wonderbra.

3. More Skin

This may hardly be noticeable to you if you are blessed with great skin tone. If you are a freckled, thin-skinned Irish lass as I am, however, the skin on your belly will fold down like a little accordion whenever you bend over at the waist. I suppose, on a dare, I could get away with wearing a two-piece bathing suit, but I would have to stay standing at attention to pull it off. I swear, you could throw a ten-carat diamond at my feet and I would not bend over to pick it up, because it would show the world my "pleats."

4. Darker Nipples

You will have noticed early on in your pregnancy that your nipples got larger and darker. After about a year postpartum, your nipples will probably have returned to their former circumference, but they will stay darker for quite some time.

5. Relaxed Vagina

Perhaps you should go pour yourself a drink before proceeding with this discussion, because my Girlfriends hate this subject almost as much as they hate the subjects of infidelity and menopause. But not talking about it doesn't make it not exist, so here goes. Once you have vaginally delivered a baby, your vagina will not ever again be as tight as it was. All of your friends who have had babies (unless they are confident and generous) will tell you that everything down there goes back to its former self, but they are just saying that because it worries them to think that their sexuality has been diminished in some way. The truth is, they are slightly looser—*and* they are probably even sexier than they were before. Experienced and fulfilled women are *always* sexier than novices.

If you have the nerve to ask your husband if he notices a difference, he will probably do some hedging or outright lying, because he undoubtedly realizes that this is an extremely sensitive topic for women. His future sex life may be completely nuked by too candid an answer. Now don't panic! You won't be left with a vagina stretched out like some old underwear elastic; you just won't be quite as firm. Your doctor knows this, even if he or she doesn't discuss it with you. That is why most of them are so willing to stitch you up nice and tight after an episiotomy; this is their idea of a consolation prize. Your husband will still want to have sex with you, and you will still enjoy it. As a matter of fact, you may enjoy it more, since your partner might now take a little longer to climax and that might give you time to catch up with him. If, however, you are not enjoying sex because your vagina feels too flaccid or feels uncomfortable for any reason, see your doctor as soon as possible, because some simple surgical procedures can easily fix this condition. There are even plastic surgeons who devote their practice to repairing this trauma. (Gasp!)

6. Lazy Bladder

Another sensation that lots of Girlfriends describe that falls into this looseness category is bladder weakness. There are degrees in this area. For example, thousands of women who have had vaginal births cannot sneeze without wetting their pants. Others say that trampoline jumping and jogging on hard surfaces present challenges their bladder can no longer meet. Then there's the situation where you just can't "hold it" the way you used to; when you have to go to the bathroom, you have to go sooner rather than later. You may also be unable to sleep an entire night without getting up to go to the bathroom. Look at it this way: This little stroll provides a nice opportunity to check on your sleeping kids and make sure they haven't kicked off their blankets.

But before you go rushing off to schedule a C-section in hopes of saving your pelvic floor, let us put things into perspective for you. Many things in life exact a toll, but they are such great experiences that we are willing to pay the price.

TOP 10
Greatest Concerns of
Pregnant Women

10. Will My Breasts Stay This Big Forever? (Please, God!)

9. Will I Feel This Sick and Tired for the Entire Nine (Ten) Months?

8. Will My Mate Ever Really Understand What I Am Going Through?

7. Will I Poop on the Delivery Table?

6. How Badly Will It Hurt to Deliver the Baby?

5. Will It Hurt More Than a Bikini Wax? Less Than a Broken Leg?

4. Will I Get All Ugly and Fat?

3. Will Everything "Down There" Shrink Back to Normal After the Baby Is Born?

2. Will I Be a Good Mother?

1. Will the Baby Be OK?

TOP 10

Reasons Why You'll Do This Again Someday

10. Mommy Alzheimer's . . . You've Already Forgotten All the Worst Parts.

9. You've Spent So Much on Baby Stuff, You Need Several More Babies to Justify the Expense.

8. It's a Good Excuse for Not Losing Those Last Fifteen Pounds, but Not *That* Good.

7. You Need Another Baby to Keep All the Grandparents from Fighting Over the One You Have.

6. You Actually Believed That Nursing Mothers Can't Get Pregnant.

5. You Are So Tired That You Can't Remember if You Inserted Your Diaphragm or Just Considered It a Good Idea.

4. You Want Those Gigantic Titties Back.

3. You Know What They Say About an Only Child.

2. An Addiction to the Intoxicating Smell Found in That Fold of Skin Right Where the Baby's Fat Little Shoulder Meets Its Neck.

1. Wine.

Index

Exercise, 61, 99–112
  clothes, 102
  compulsion to, 108–109
  danger to pregnancy, 104–106
  Kegels, 110–12
  labor and delivery, 103–104
  postpartum weight loss and, 106–108
  reasons not to, 100–109
  relaxation and flexibility, 109–10
  tiredness and, 100–101
Exhaustion. *See* Fatigue
Expectations about birth experience, 76,
    219–20, 233

Face:
  acne, 35
  hair, 37, 148
  pigmentation, 37, 140–41, 149
  swelling, 28, 32
False labor, myth of, 217–19
Fashion, 127–51
  bathing suits, 138–41
  bras, 143–46, 151
  celebration of belly, 128–30
  challenges, 132–46
  costs, 137
  designer, 128
  fabrics, 127–28, 133
  girdles and panty hose, 141–43
  going-home outfit, 192–93
  panties, 141
  scratching and, 133
  sharing with pregnant girlfriends, 137–38,
    150
  temperature fluctuations, 132–33
  vaginal and breast secretions, 132–33
  weight gain and, 134–37
  what to bring to hospital, 191–93
  at work, 130–32
  yoga, 130
Father, 11–12, 153–63
  baby delivered by, 160
  blaming, 60
  as birth coach, 156–58, 230
  communication gap, 154–55
  fears of, 158–63
  gift for wife in hospital, 195
  his own father and, 162–63
  irrational feelings toward, 58–60
  need to be mothered, 158–59
  obstetrician choice and, 76–77
  postpartum sex and, 161, 243–46,
    252–53

sharing pregnancy news with, 13–16
sharing pregnancy news with your father,
    19–20
sympathy symptoms of (couvade
    syndrome), 59–60, 155–56
See also Partner
Fatigue, 2–3
  in early pregnancy, 2–3, 100
  exercise and, 100–101
  postpartum, 244–45
Fears, 109
  about newborns, 237–40
  irrational, 60–72
Feet, 137, 183
  postpartum, 251
Fetal monitor, 227
Fiber, 47
Financial worries, 159
First pregnancy, 11, 12, 28, 184, 228
First wife, comparisons with, 67
Flatulence, 39–40
Folic acid, 45
Food, 5, 58, 107
  balanced diet, 6
  comfort, 5–6
  cravings, 46, 57–58, 59
  early labor and, 218–19
  for hospital, 197–98
  immediate gratification, 57–58
  last month of pregnancy, 181, 187
  morning sickness and, 4–6, 42–43, 45
  sensitivities, 4–6
  spicy, 187
Forgetfulness, 54–55
Freckles, 149

Gas, 39–40
Gender of baby, 43, 63, 87–88, 109,
    233–34
  morning sickness and, 43
Genetics, 34–35
  miscarriage and, 61
  tests, 63, 89–95, 170–71
Girdles, 141–43
Girlfriends, 17
  at labor and delivery, 158, 201–202
  sharing pregnancy news with, 17
Glucose tolerance test, 88–89
Going-home outfit, 192–93
Gonal F, 165
Grandfathers, 19–20
Grandmothers, 17–19
Guilt, 63